An Atlas of
Gross
Pathology

Christopher DM Fletcher MB BS MRCPath

Lecturer and Honorary Senior Registrar in Histopathology
St. Thomas's Hospital Medical School, London, UK

Phillip H McKee MB BCh BaO MRCPath

Senior Lecturer and Honorary Consultant in Histopathology
St. Thomas's Hospital Medical School, London, UK

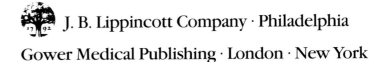

J. B. Lippincott Company · Philadelphia

Gower Medical Publishing · London · New York

Distributed in USA and Canada by:
J. B. Lippincott Company
East Washington Square
Philadelphia, PA 19105
USA

Distributed in Japan by:
Nankodo Company Limited
42-6 Hongo 3-chome
Bunkyo, Tokyo 113
Japan

**Distributed in all countries except
USA, Canada and Japan by:**
Edward Arnold
A Division of Hodder and Stoughton
LONDON   MELBOURNE   AUCKLAND

British Library Cataloguing in Publication Data:

Fletcher, Christopher D.M.
   An atlas of gross pathology.
   1. Pathology
   I. Title II. McKee, Phillip H.
   616.07   RB111

ISBN: 0-7131-4557-9 (Arnold)
      0-397-44607-1 (Lippincott)

Library of Congress Catalog Number: 89-85558

Project Editor: Michele Campbell
Design: Nigel Duffield
Illustration: Pamela Corfield

Set in Garamond and Helvetica by:
Informat Computer Communications Ltd.

Originated in Hong Kong by:
Imago Publishing Ltd.

Reprinted in Singapore in 1989 by:
Imago Productions (FE) PTE Limited.

Print number 8 7 6 5 4 3 2 1

Preface

The aim of this atlas is to provide an introduction to the macroscopical appearances of the most common pathological conditions for undergraduate medical students and nurses in training. It will also, hopefully, be of value to postgraduates undertaking the FRCS examinations, for whom a working knowledge of gross pathology is vital.

Only important or frequently encountered disease processes are covered. Each illustration is accompanied by a concise legend outlining basic, relevant clinicopathological and pathogenetic details. In collecting material for this atlas, we are deeply indebted to Professor J.R. Tighe of the Histopathology Department at St. Thomas's Hospital for allowing us access to the departmental collection of colour transparencies. We are also particularly grateful to Dr H. Pambakian, Museum Curator at St. Thomas's Hospital Medical School and Professors H. Spencer and M.S.R. Hutt. Most of all, this book would not have been possible without the consistent generosity and thoughtfulness of all the pathologists in our department, who unselfishly offered us many of their specimens, obtained either surgically or at post mortem, for photography.

CDM Fletcher & PH McKee
London

Acknowledgements

The authors would like to thank the following colleagues for providing illustrative material: Professor P.G. Bullough, Cornell University Medical College, New York (Figs.7.16, 12.1 bottom, 12.4, 12.7-12.10, 12.13-12.15, 12.17, 12.18, 12.20-22, 12.24, 12.25 & 12.29 top); Dr D.W. Day, Dept. of Pathology, University of Liverpool Medical School, Liverpool (Fig.3.23); Dr C.W. Elston, Dept. of Pathology, City Hospital, Nottingham (Fig.9.35); Professor P.L. Lantos, Dept. of Neuropathology, Institute of Psychiatry, London (Figs.11.10, 11.20 & 11.24); Dr J.C. Macartney, Dept. of Histopathology, St Thomas's Hospital Medical School, London (Figs.4.26, 4.29, 7.8 & 12.26); Professor F.V. O'Brien, School of Dentistry, Queen's University, Belfast (Figs.3.1 & 3.2); Dr C. Parkinson, Institute of Urology, London (Figs.10.7 & 10.13); Dr D.E. Sharvill, William Harvey Hospital, Ashford, Kent (Fig.5.13); Dr J.M. Sloan, Senior Lecturer/Consultant Pathologist, Royal Victoria Hospital, Belfast (Figs.2.3, 2.4, 2.14, 8.24 & 8.30); The Wellcome Museum, Royal College of Surgeons of England, London (Figs.8.20 & 9.28).

Contents

1 Cardiovascular System

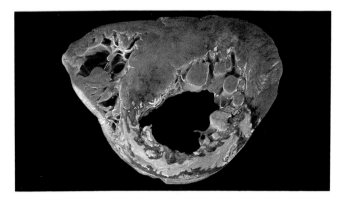

Fig.1.1 Recent myocardial infarct. A transverse section through both right and left ventricles, viewed from below. The anterior wall of the left ventricle shows an extensive area of recent infarction, characterised by an almost full-thickness zone of yellow necrotic myocardium, surrounded by a hyperaemic rim. The latter consists of granulation tissue (capillaries and fibroblasts) and represents the early phase of healing. This infarct is of approximately one week's duration. In nearly all cases, myocardial infarction is caused by occlusive thrombosis in an atheromatous coronary artery. Rare causes include syphilitic aortitis, polyarteritis nodosa and coronary artery embolism from a variety of cardiac lesions.

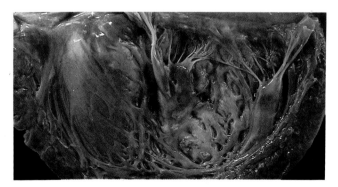

Fig.1.2 Healed myocardial infarct. The heart has been opened to display the inner aspect of the left ventricle. Marked pale fibrous scarring is seen in the posterior wall and in the papillary muscles. Mural thrombus overlying the scar is also present. Healing, by fibrosis, commences about 3 weeks after acute infarction and is usually complete after 2 months. Fibrous replacement of the myocardium predisposes to aneurysm formation (see Fig.1.6) within which thrombus may form.

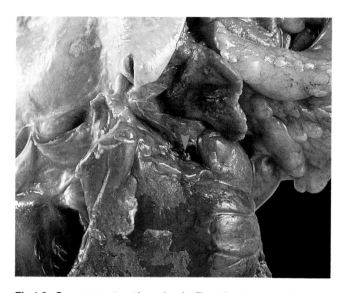

Fig.1.3 Coronary artery thrombosis. The left main stem coronary artery has been opened longitudinally to reveal occlusion of its lumen by thrombus (arrowed). Note the presence of atheroma in the ascending aorta and a fibrinous pericarditis. Occlusive coronary thrombosis almost always occurs at the site of an atheromatous stenosis (see Figs.1.36-1.38) and is thought to be initiated either by ulceration or haemorrhage into a plaque.

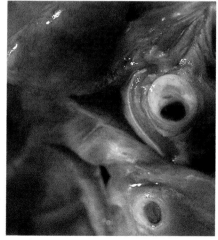

Fig.1.4 Coronary artery thrombosis. The left anterior descending coronary artery is shown in transverse section. The lumen is markedly diminished by atheroma, and overlying thrombus has resulted in total occlusion. In the vast majority of cases of myocardial infarction, such occlusive thrombosis will be detected if the coronary arteries are examined with sufficient care.

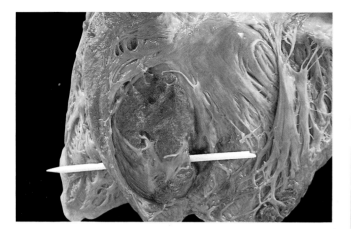

Fig.1.5 Myocardial infarct with mural thrombus and ventricular rupture. The heart has been opened to expose the septal wall of the left ventricle. A large mural thrombus is adherent to an area of recent myocardial infarction, complicated by rupture of the interventricular septum. The probe has been passed through the rupture and at the extreme left of the picture its tip can be seen overlying the right ventricular flap. Myocardial rupture, which is not uncommon, usually occurs within a week of acute infarction.

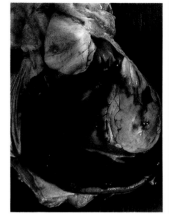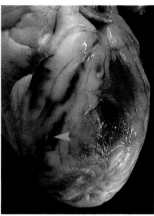

Fig.1.7 Haemopericardium. The pericardial sac has been opened (left) to show an extensive haematoma overlying the epicardium. On the right, the haematoma has been removed to reveal the cause as being a slit-like ventricular perforation (arrowed) at the site of a recent myocardial infarct. Haemopericardium may more rarely occur as a complication of dissecting aortic aneurysm or trauma.

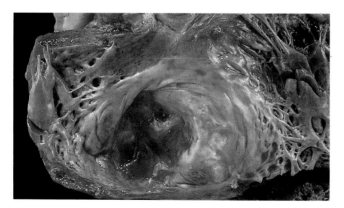

Fig.1.6 Left ventricular aneurysm. The development of an aneurysm of the left ventricle is a not uncommon late complication of myocardial infarction. It is due to replacement of the myocardium by collagenous scar tissue with resultant loss of elasticity. Such aneurysms often contain mural thrombus which may be a source of systemic emboli. The laceration of the anterior papillary muscle to the right of the aneurysm occurred during the post mortem.

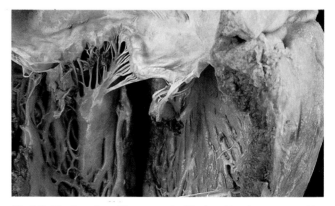

Fig.1.8 Ruptured papillary muscle. The heart has been opened to display the posterior aspect of the left ventricle. In the centre of the picture is a portion of the anterior papillary muscle which has been torn and shows obvious necrosis. Rupture of a papillary muscle is a rare complication of myocardial infarction, which usually occurs within 2 weeks of the primary event: it results in the acute onset of mitral incompetence and left ventricular failure.

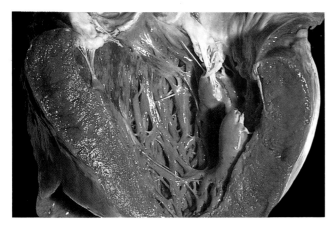

Fig.1.9 Left ventricular hypertrophy. Left ventricular hypertrophy is a not uncommon finding at post mortem owing to the frequency of essential hypertension in the population. A list of causes is given in Fig.1.10. In this instance the increased thickness of the left ventricular wall is obvious (in excess of 20mm). However, a much more accurate method of assessing ventricular hypertrophy involves weighing the chambers separately after careful dissection, thereby taking into account any degree of associated ventricular dilatation.

CAUSES OF LEFT VENTRICULAR HYPERTROPHY	
Systemic hypertension	
Aortic stenosis	
Aortic incompetence	
Mitral incompetence	
Congenital heart disease	coarctation of aorta
	reversed VSD
Amyloid	
Cardiomyopathy	
High output failure	anaemia
	thyrotoxicosis
	Paget's disease
	A-V malformation

Fig.1.10 Causes of left ventricular hypertrophy.

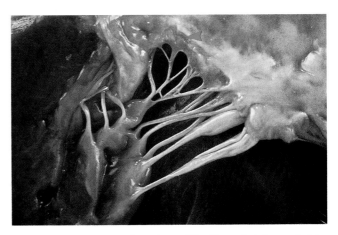

Fig.1.11 Acute rheumatic endocarditis. Characteristic small pink vegetations (arrowed) are present along the line of closure of this mitral valve cusp. Rheumatic fever, a multisystem autoimmune process, is a rare complication of β-haemolytic (Group A) streptococcal infections. It results from the development of heterophilic cross-reacting antibodies to the streptococcal M protein and an, as yet unidentified, connective tissue antigen. Manifestations include a pancarditis, joint involvement, skin rashes, subcutaneous nodules and, rarely, Sydenham's chorea.

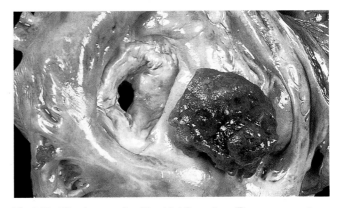

Fig.1.12 Mitral stenosis with atrial thrombus. The commonest complication of rheumatic endocarditis is mitral stenosis and, indeed, almost all stenotic mitral valves are of rheumatic origin. Fusion of the valve cusps and fibrosis results in narrowing of the valve orifice. The stenosis causes left atrial dilatation and may be complicated by atrial fibrillation with consequent thrombus formation, as seen in this case.

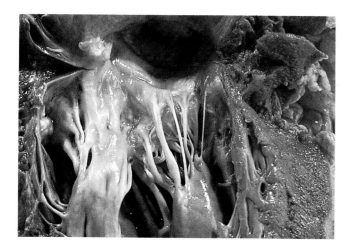

Fig.1.13 Mixed mitral valve disease. There is marked fibrosis of the chordae tendinae with fusion and shortening. The rheumatic process has produced a rigid 'buttonhole' valve, thereby being both stenotic and incompetent - the latter has resulted in the development of left ventricular hypertrophy, as seen in the bottom right hand corner.

CAUSES OF MITRAL INCOMPETENCE
Rheumatic heart disease
Papillary muscle rupture or fibrosis
Congenital
Mitral valve prolapse (floppy valve syndrome)
Functional dilatation of valve ring
Marfan's syndrome

Fig.1.14 Causes of mitral incompetence.

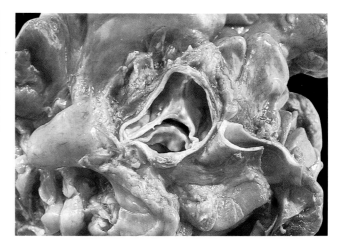

Fig.1.15 Aortic stenosis. Isolated aortic stenosis may complicate rheumatic heart disease but more often is associated with mitral involvement also. The proximal portion of the ascending aorta has been opened to view this stenotic valve from above. Aortic stenosis usually gives rise to left ventricular hypertrophy and may compromise the coronary blood supply.

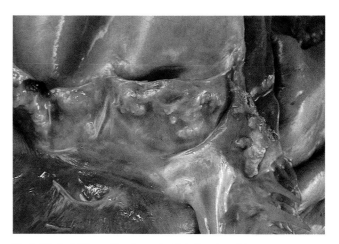

Fig.1.16 Calcific aortic stenosis. Calcification of the aortic valve most commonly occurs in a congenital bicuspid valve, but may also arise as a consequence of rheumatic disease and is sometimes a feature of the ageing process. Note the coarse calcific nodules in the valve cusps.

CAUSES OF AORTIC STENOSIS		
Rheumatic heart disease		
Calcification	of congenital bicuspid valve	
	senile	
Congenital	dome-shaped valve	
	supravalvar stenosis	
	subvalvar stenosis	
Hypertrophic cardiomyopathy		

Fig.1.17 Causes of aortic stenosis.

CAUSES OF AORTIC INCOMPETENCE
Rheumatic heart disease
Syphilitic aortitis
Congenital bicuspid valve
Marfan's syndrome
Ankylosing spondylitis
Aortic sinus aneurysm

Fig.1.18 Causes of aortic incompetence.

TYPES OF ENDOCARDITIS		
Infective		bacterial
		viral
		rickettsial
		chlamydial
		fungal
Rheumatic		
Non-infective thrombotic (agonal)		
Libman-Sacks (S.L.E.)		

Fig.1.19 Types of endocarditis.

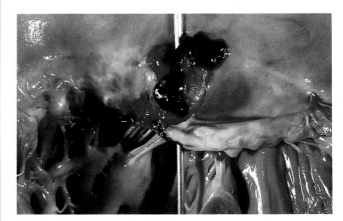

Fig.1.20 Infective endocarditis (damaged valve). Infection of the endocardium and valves may be due to a diverse variety of micro-organisms (Fig.1.19) and, while it may affect previously normal tissue, it develops more often in the presence of pre-existing (particularly rheumatic) valvular disease. *Streptococcus viridans* is the commonest cause of infective endocarditis in previously damaged valves but *Staphylococcus aureus*, β-haemolytic Streptococci and *Streptococcus pneumoniae* are the most usual aetiological agents in cases with no evidence of prior disease. Large friable vegetations obscure the underlying fibrosed mitral valve in this case.

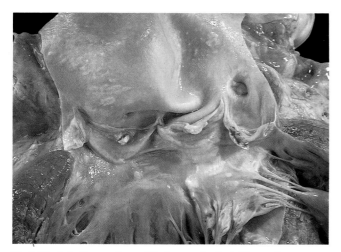

Fig.1.21 Infective endocarditis (normal valve). Vegetations are present on all three cusps of this otherwise normal aortic valve. Endocarditis affecting normal valves is usually a more fulminant disease affecting immunocompromised patients and drug addicts: in the latter group the right side of the heart may be involved.

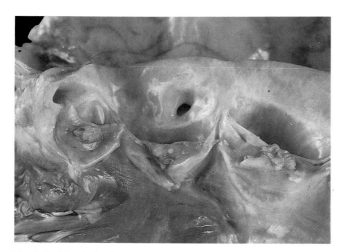

Fig.1.22 Non-infective thrombotic endocarditis. This condition, which may affect the aortic and mitral valves, is often found in patients dying with disseminated malignant tumours. The pink vegetations seen on this aortic valve are similar to, and may be confused with, those of rheumatic endocarditis.

TYPES OF CARDIOMYOPATHY	
Hypertrophic (± obstruction)	
Congestive, may be associated with	alcoholism
	parturition
	beri-beri
	Friedreich's ataxia
	muscular dystrophies
Restrictive (endomyocardial fibroelastosis)	
Obliterative (endomyocardial fibrosis)	
Löffler's endocarditis	

Fig.1.23 Types of cardiomyopathy.

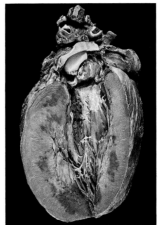

Fig.1.24 Hypertrophic obstructive cardiomyopathy. A true cardiomyopathy is, by definition, any myocardial disease without an identifiable cause which appears non-inflammatory. Hypertrophic cardiomyopathy is typified by asymmetrical left ventricular hypertrophy, especially of the septal wall. Most commonly it is familial, the mode of inheritance being autosomal dominant. In this case the septal hypertrophy has led to obstruction of the out-flow tract. Hypertrophic obstructive cardiomyopathy is a rare but important cause of unexpected sudden death.

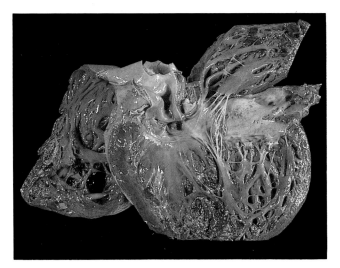

Fig.1.25 Congestive cardiomyopathy. Congestive cardio-myopathy is defined as congestive cardiac failure with no apparent cause, and results in a dilated, flabby heart, as in this case. This appearance may be seen in association with alcohol abuse and pregnancy.

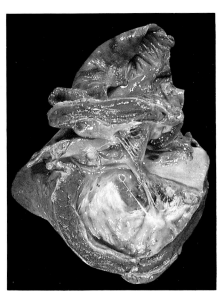

Fig.1.26 Endo-myocardial fibrosis. Endomyo-cardial fibrosis occurs most commonly in tropical Africans and is manifest as dense fibrosis of the ventricular endocardium. A popular hypothesis is that the lesion has a viral aetiology. Involvement of the papillary muscles may induce valve dysfunction.

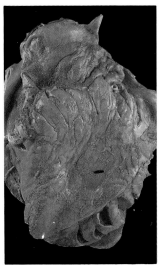

Fig.1.27 Fibrinous pericarditis. Pericarditis may occasionally be due to primary pyogenic infection, but more commonly a fibrinous exudate occurs as a consequence of a variety of disorders including myocardial infarction (Fig.1.3), rheumatic fever, uraemia, connective tissue diseases and adjacent infective conditions, for example bacterial pneumonia (in which instance the exudate may be fibrinopurulent). In this case a generalised septicaemia has resulted in a typical 'bread and butter' appearance.

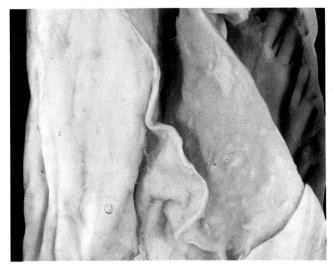

Fig.1.28 Tuberculous pericarditis. The adherent parietal and visceral pericardial membranes have been separated to display numerous small white miliary tubercles on the surface of the latter. Note also the pale fibrous thickening of the parietal layer. Tuberculous pericarditis is said to result from lymphatic spread of organisms from adjacent pulmonary or mediastinal foci of infection.

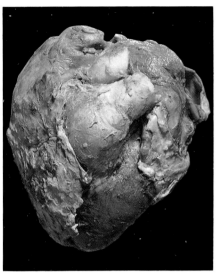

Fig.1.29 Constrictive pericarditis. This is a very rare disease in which the heart becomes encased by a densely adherent, thickened and fibrotic pericardium. The aetiology is often uncertain. While some cases may be due to tuberculous infection, occasionally a collagen disease is implicated.

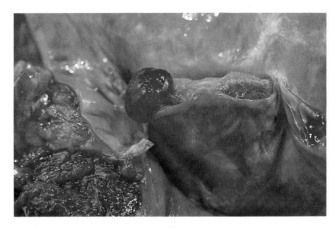

Fig.1.31 Lambl's excrescence. The occurrence of small fibrin deposits on the heart valves is not an uncommon finding at post mortem. Occasionally they may acquire tumour-like appearances, as seen in this case. The aetiology is uncertain.

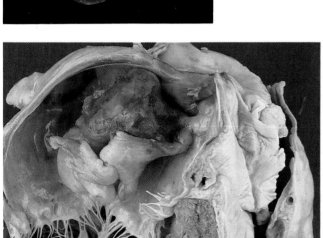

Fig.1.30 Left atrial myxoma. The heart has been opened to display the left atrium and mitral valve. Attached to the posterior wall of the left atrium is a large, pedunculated multilobular tumour. Atrial myxomas are rare and clinically may present with multiple systemic emboli, or occasionally, with acute pulmonary oedema due to obstruction of the mitral valve orifice. Their precise nature is, as yet, uncertain since there is argument as to whether they represent true neoplasms or are simply organised thrombi.

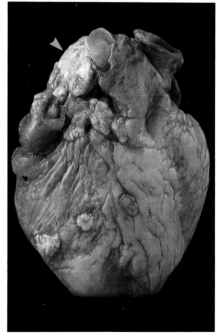

Fig.1.32 Epicardial secondary deposits. This heart was taken from an elderly male dying from squamous cell carcinoma of the bronchus. The epicardium is covered by small pale umbilicated metastases. In addition there is a large tumour mass situated between the superior vena cava and the pulmonary trunk, seen at the top of the picture (arrowed). This resulted in vena caval obstruction. Epicardial or pericardial tumour metastases often induce a fibrinous or fibrinopurulent pericarditis.

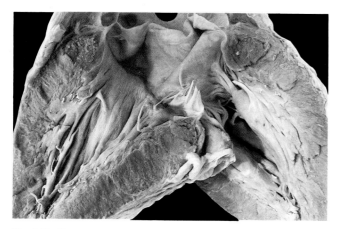

Fig.1.33 Brown atrophy. This heart, which was removed from an 86-year-old woman with senile dementia, is very small and weighed only 180g (normal adult female 250-300g). Note the brownish discolouration. This change is an ageing phenomenon, in which lipofuscin pigment, representing the lipid remnants of effete organelles, is deposited in many organs in association with atrophic changes, probably due to a combination of relative ischaemia and disuse.

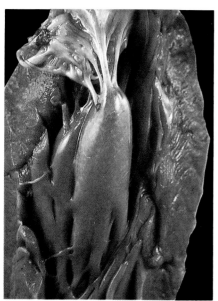

Fig.1.34 Myocardial fatty degeneration. Accumulation of lipid within the myocardium may occur in a variety of conditions including severe anaemia, alcohol abuse and poisoning. As seen in this papillary muscle, it produces a characteristic 'thrush breast' appearance.

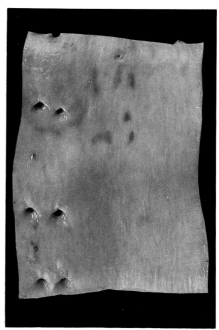

Fig.1.35 Fatty streaks (aorta). This aorta has been removed from a small child and stained by the Oil Red O technique to demonstrate lipid. Small intimal deposits are seen. The orifices of the intercostal arteries are on the left. Such juvenile fatty streaks are found in the large arteries of children and adolescents of all races and socio-economic groups. It is unlikely that these lesions bear any pathogenetic relationship to the future development of atheromatous plaques.

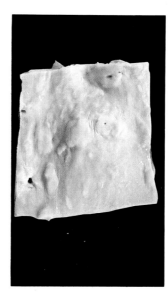

Fig.1.36 Uncomplicated atheroma. This section of aorta, from a middle-aged male, shows numerous raised, irregular intimal deposits. Atheroma is the commonest cause of death in the Western World, largely by giving rise to myocardial infarction and cerebrovascular accidents. Known risk factors for its development include increasing age, cigarette smoking, hypertension, a diet high in saturated fats, hyperlipidaemia and diabetes mellitus. Its exact pathogenesis is unclear, but intra-intimal lipid deposition and incorporation of mural thrombi are popular hypotheses. Myofibroblasts within plaques have been shown to be monoclonal in origin, the significance of which is uncertain.

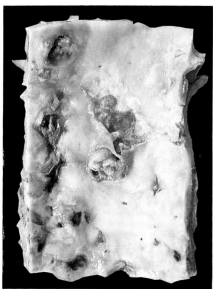

Fig.1.37 Ulcerated atheroma. Necrosis within an atheromatous plaque, in combination with constant haemodynamic stress may lead to ulceration, as seen in this picture. As a consequence, exposure of subendothelial tissues may result in thrombus formation. This in turn may cause vascular occlusion of medium and small arteries, as seen in the coronary vessels (Figs.1.3 and 1.4).

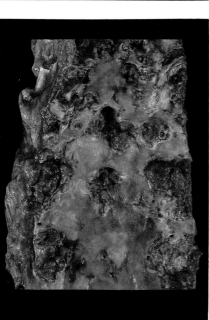

Fig.1.38 Complicated atheroma. This segment of aorta has been opened to show all the major complications that may occur in atheromatous plaques. There is extensive ulceration, haemorrhage and dystrophic calcification; scattered small thrombi are present, overlying some of the lesions. It is not uncommon for fragments of such complicated plaques to break off and produce systemic emboli, the consequences of which will clearly depend on the site of the affected artery.

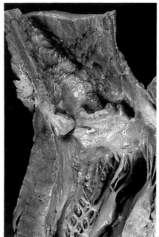

Fig.1.39 Syphilitic aortitis. The left ventricle and ascending aorta have been opened to show the characteristic irregular 'wood bark' appearance of the aortic intima. The aortic valve cusps are rolled and thickened and there is separation of the commissures. Syphilitic aortitis is the commonest manifestation of tertiary infection and usually affects only the intrathoracic portion of the aorta. It results from a florid arteritis of the vasa vasorum with consequent intimal fibrosis. Common complications of this condition include aortic incompetence, aneurysm formation and stenosis of the ostia of the coronary arteries.

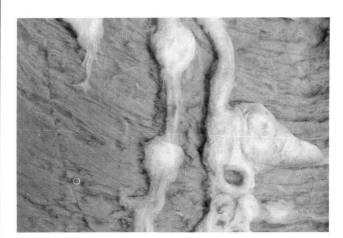

Fig.1.40 Polyarteritis nodosa. The epicardium has been stripped from this heart to demonstrate branches of one of the coronary arteries, which show fibrosis of the vessel walls and formation of several small saccular aneurysms. Polyarteritis nodosa is an uncommon disease, thought to be due to immune complex deposition and sometimes associated with hepatitis B or systemic lupus erythematosus. It affects small arteries and arterioles in any part of the body and results in inflammation and necrosis of the vessel walls, commonly with overlying thrombosis. The clinical effects are largely due to ischaemia of the affected organs. Small aneurysms develop quite often and may be complicated by rupture.

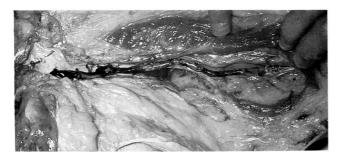

Fig.1.41 Deep venous thrombosis. The femoral vein has been exposed in a patient dying of pulmonary embolism (see Fig.2.16). The lumen of the vein is virtually occluded by thrombus which is adherent to the endothelial surface. In general terms the predisposing factors to thrombosis are encompassed in Virchow's triad: (1) alteration in the vessel wall, (2) alteration in the blood flow and (3) alteration in the blood constituents. Deep venous thrombosis is commonest in the calf veins and, as in this case, may be complicated by pulmonary embolism, although the frequency with which this occurs is difficult to determine since many venous thromboses go undetected. The commonest causes include immobility, myocardial infarction, pregnancy or childbirth, varicose veins or phlebitis and any severely debilitating disease such as cancer.

CLASSIFICATION OF TRUE ANEURYSMS
Atheromatous
Syphilitic
Infective
Cirsoid
A-V fistula
Berry (cerebral)
Charcot-Bouchard (cerebral-hypertensive)
Erdheim's medial degeneration (dissecting)
Marfan's disease (dissecting)

Fig.1.42 Types of true aneurysm, to be distinguished from a 'false' aneurysm, which represents the site of a walled-off arterial rupture.

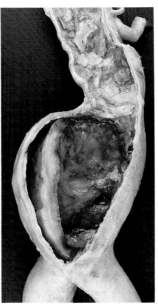

Fig.1.43 Abdominal aortic aneurysm. The lower portion of the abdominal aorta has been opened to show a saccular dilation of the distal end, the lumen of which contains a large laminated thrombus. Proximally, the aorta shows extensive involvement by complicated atheroma. This is the commonest variety of true aortic aneurysm in the Western World and is almost always a consequence of extensive atheroma, leading to thinning or disruption of the aortic media. Older adults, particularly males, are often affected. Such aneurysms may rupture with extensive retroperitoneal haemorrhage and this may be fatal. The formation of large intraluminal thrombi sometimes gives rise to aortic occlusion with distal ischaemia or to embolic phenomena.

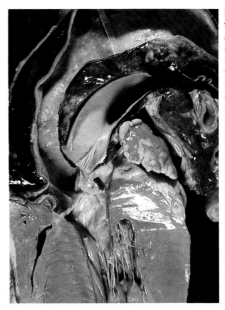

Fig.1.44 Dissecting aortic aneurysm. The term dissecting aneurysm is a misnomer in that true dilatation of the vessel wall does not occur. Rather, the apparent increase in size is due to the presence of thrombus within the media of the artery, as seen here in the arch of the aorta. Dissecting aneurysm is most commonly due to mucoid degeneration (Erdheim) of the media but may also be seen in Marfan's syndrome and in association with systemic hypertension.

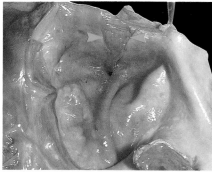

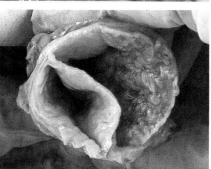

Fig.1.45 Dissecting aortic aneurysm. The process of dissection is initiated by a transverse intimal tear (arrowed), usually in the proximal part of the ascending aorta (top). Extension of the process causes formation of a false lumen within the media which, on transverse section, produces a typical double-barrelled appearance (bottom). Dissecting aneurysm is usually fatal either by rupture or by retrograde involvement of the coronary arteries. Very occasionally the dissecting process re-enters the true lumen of the aorta.

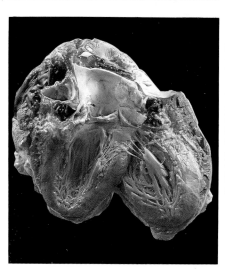

Fig.1.46 Dissecting aortic aneurysm. In this instance the dissection has resulted in rupture of the aortic root and the development of haemopericardium. External rupture may also occur into the pleural cavity (leading to a haemothorax) or mediastinum.

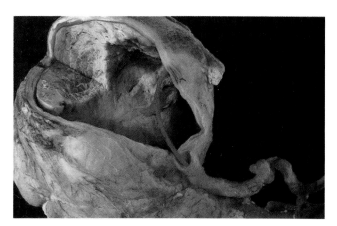

Fig.1.47 Splenic artery aneurysm. The large saccular aneurysm above the body of the pancreas was found in a young woman with no evidence of atheroma or syphilis. The red probe demonstrates luminal continuity between the aneurysm and the distal portion of the artery. The lesion probably represents a rare example of a congenital aneurysm due to fibromuscular displasia of the arterial wall.

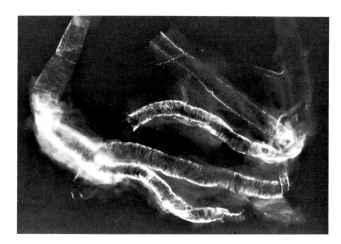

Fig.1.48 Mönckeberg's sclerosis. Mönckeberg's sclerosis is characterised by calcification of the media of the large arteries, particularly in the limbs and pelvis. It appears to be part of the normal ageing process and is commoner in diabetics. The diagnosis is usually made radiologically. In this plain X-ray of a post-mortem specimen of the femoral arteries, the typical fine tram-line appearance of the calcification is clearly seen.

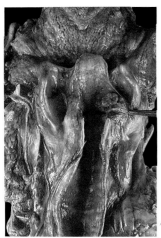

Fig.2.1 Laryngeal squamous carcinoma. The trachea and larynx have been opened posteriorly to reveal a small fungating supraglottic tumour arising in the right aryepiglottic fold. Squamous carcinoma is the commonest malignant tumour of the larynx and arises most often in the 6th and 7th decades, affecting males more frequently than females. Known risk factors include chronic inflammation and cigarette smoking. Spread is largely local or lymphatic and overall 5-year survival is about 65%.

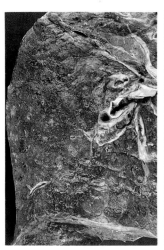 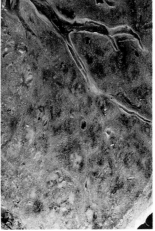

Fig.2.2 Bronchopneumonia. This left lung shows congestion and diffuse multifocal consolidation (left). A close-up view from a different case (right) shows small areas of consolidation and suppuration, largely centrilobular in distribution. Bronchopneumonia is principally a disease of the very young and old, but also occurs in immunosuppressed patients. Chronic obstructive airways disease and viral respiratory infections are frequent predisposing factors. A very wide variety of causative organisms may be isolated, of which *Streptococcus pneumoniae*, *Streptococcus pyogenes* and *Haemophilus influenzae* are the most frequent.

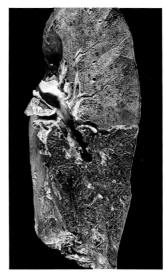

Fig.2.3 Lobar pneumonia. Uniform red, firm consolidation of this left upper lobe, with complete sparing of the lower lobe, is typical of 'red hepatisation' - the second stage of lobar pneumonia. This occurs at about the 2nd to 4th days in an untreated patient, being preceded by engorgement and succeeded by 'grey hepatisation' and resolution at about the 8th to 10th day. Lobar pneumonia, particularly in its classical form, is rarely seen nowadays with the advent of modern antibiotic therapy. However, young adults are often affected, over 90% of cases being due to *Streptococcus pneumoniae*.

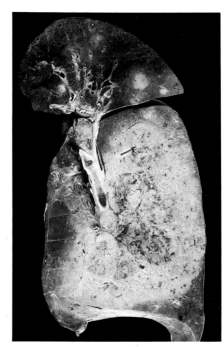

Fig.2.4 Lobar pneumonia. There is a fairly uniform 'grey hepatisation' of the left lower lobe with five small foci of consolidation in the upper lobe adjacent to the oblique fissure. This appearance is due to the massive influx of inflammatory cells, associated with relative ischaemia. Complications of lobar pneumonia include the development of septicaemia, an empyema, a lung abscess or carnification (extensive fibrosis).

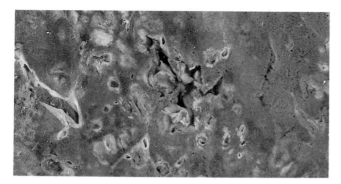

Fig.2.5 Staphylococcal pneumonia. A close-up view of this lung shows numerous characteristic foci of centrilobular suppuration which, in the upper centre, have coalesced to form a small pulmonary abscess. Staphylococcal pneumonia most often complicates viral infections or is nosocomial in origin. Suppuration and abscess formation are similarly seen in Klebsiella pneumonia, which may also be a hospital-acquired infection. Both carry a relatively high mortality and, in those who survive, extensive lung damage may remain.

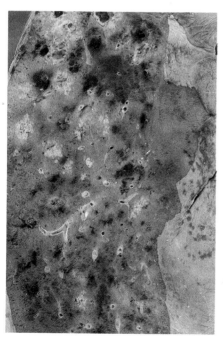

Fig.2.6 Aspiration pneumonia. The apex of this lower lobe shows multiple small foci of pale consolidation with microabscess formation principally localised around the smaller airways. Aspiration pneumonia follows inhalation of material from the oropharynx, oesophagus or stomach and is commonest in unconscious patients, alcoholics and those with an upper alimentary obstructive lesion. Aspiration of sterile gastric secretions is known as Mendelson's syndrome.

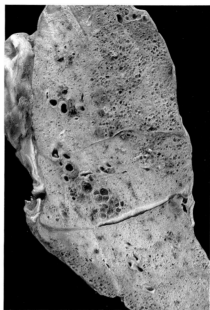

Fig.2.7 Lipid pneumonia. This lung shows uniform pale, rather waxy, consolidation. Note also the pre-existent bronchiectasis and centriacinar emphysema. Lipid pneumonia may either be exogenous, due to inhalation of ingested or regurgitated oils taken in medication or food, or may be endogenous, occurring most often distal to an obstructing bronchial carcinoma and resulting from excessive accumulation of surfactant.

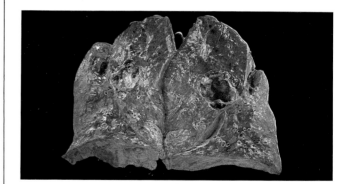

Fig.2.8 Lung abscess. This lung has been hemisected to show a large necrotic abscess cavity in the upper lobe. Note also the marked congestion and pre-existent bronchiectasis. Lung abscess is most often due to infection by Staphylococci, Klebsiella or Pneumococcus Type 3. It may develop after inhalation of foreign material or result from a septic embolus. Such abscesses are commonest in the upper lobes and may be complicated by rupture into a bronchus or the pleural cavity, pleurisy or extensive lung scarring. Alternatively, they may become walled-off and resolve.

CAUSES OF BRONCHIECTASIS

CONGENITAL	Mucoviscidosis	
	Bronchial malformation	
ACQUIRED	Pulmonary infection	unresolved bronchitis or pneumonia
		viral lung infections
	Bronchial obstruction	tumour
		hilar lymph nodes (especially TB)
		foreign body

Fig.2.9 Causes of bronchiectasis.

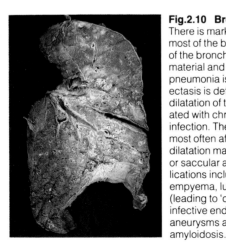

Fig.2.10 Bronchiectasis. There is marked dilatation of most of the bronchial tree. Many of the bronchi contain purulent material and extensive broncho-pneumonia is present. Bronchi-ectasis is defined as irreversible dilatation of the bronchi associ-ated with chronic suppurative infection. The lower lobes are most often affected and areas of dilatation may assume a fusiform or saccular appearance. Comp-lications include lung abscess, empyema, lung damage (leading to 'cor pulmonale'), infective endocarditis, mycotic aneurysms and secondary amyloidosis.

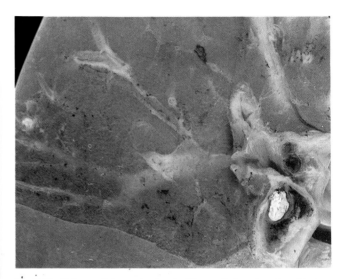

Fig.2.11 Primary tuberculosis. Just beneath the pleural surface (left) is a small, pale nodule (Ghon focus): the hilar lymph nodes show fibrosis and calcification. The combination of these two lesions is known as a primary complex, which in this case is resolving. Primary pulmonary tuberculosis remains endemic in underdeveloped countries and is almost always caused by *Mycobacterium tuberculosis*. Children or young adults are most often affected. Most lesions heal spontaneously, but progressive infection with abscess formation, bronchopneumonia or miliary spread may occur.

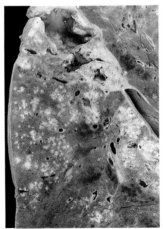

Fig.2.12 Post-primary tuberculosis. In the apex of this lower lobe, there is an irregular cavity, containing caseous material, which has ruptured into a bronchus resulting in intra-pulmonary bronchopneumonic spread. Post-primary tuber-culosis is far more often due to exogenous reinfection than reactivation of previous endo-genous infection. The lobar apices are typically affected and other complications of cavitation include spread to the upper res-piratory or alimentary tracts. Secondary amyloidosis may develop in long-standing cases.

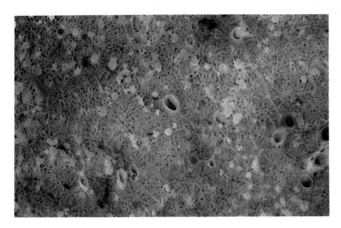

Fig.2.13 Miliary tuberculosis. Throughout the lung parenchyma, and particularly numerous around blood vessels, are small discrete 'tubercles'. Miliary spread is due to haematogenous dissemination of Mycobacteria and may complicate either primary infection (in which destructive foci erode into blood vessels) or reactivated post-primary infection in debilitated, elderly patients.

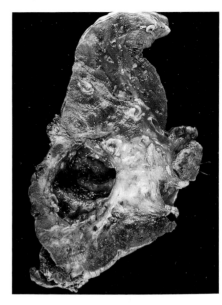

Fig.2.15 Cavitating tuberculosis. This is an upper lobectomy specimen which contains a ragged, haemorrhagic cavity extending just beneath the visceral pleura. The cavity is surrounded by an area of pale caseous necrosis. Such an appearance may represent progressive primary or, more commonly, post-primary infection and results from liquefaction of caseous material.

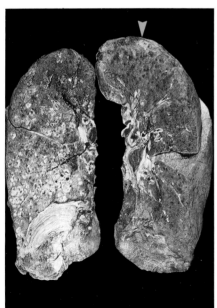

Fig.2.14 Tuberculous bronchopneumonia. The right lung shows multiple foci of caseous pneumonia. At the apex of the left lung a small subpleural area of scarring and caseation is apparent (arrowed). Tuberculous bronchopneumonia typically complicates post-primary (reinfection) disease and results from the intrabronchial spread of the liquefied contents of a caseous cavity.

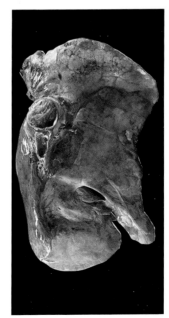

Fig.2.16 Pulmonary embolism. The right main pulmonary artery is virtually occluded by a massive laminated thrombus. The lung is rather pale in appearance. Pulmonary embolism most often complicates deep venous thromboses in the lower limb (see Fig. 1.41). The commonest predisposing factors are prolonged bed rest, particularly after surgical operations, parturition, congestive cardiac failure and hypercoagulability. Massive emboli, such as the one shown here, prevent the passage of blood into the pulmonary circulation and result in sudden death. Smaller emboli, which lodge in more distal vessels, may have no effect, or may result in pulmonary hypertension and cause infarction (see Fig. 2.17) or may give rise to pulmonary haemosiderosis.

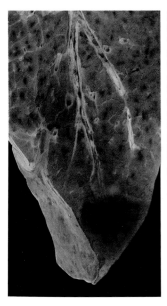

Fig.2.17 Pulmonary infarct. At the tip of the lower lobe is a wedge-shaped area of typical, dark-red infarction. Proximally, two branches of the pulmonary artery are occluded by embolic thrombus. Pulmonary infarcts are commonest in late adulthood and are predominantly a complication of deep venous thrombosis (see Fig. 1.41). Most pulmonary infarcts are of the 'red' congested type as true ischaemic necrosis is prevented by the dual blood supply from the bronchial artery.

CAUSES OF PULMONARY HAEMOSIDEROSIS	
Pulmonary hypertension	chronic left ventricular failure
	mitral valve disease
	left atrial myxoma
Goodpasture's syndrome	
Long-standing haemochromatosis	
Haemosiderosis	

Fig.2.18 Causes of pulmonary haemosiderosis.

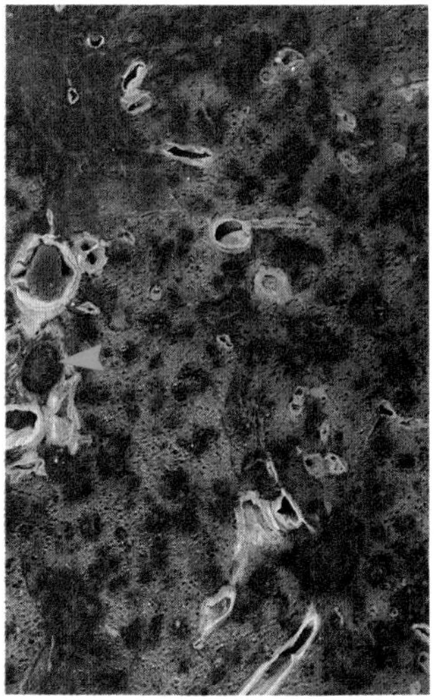

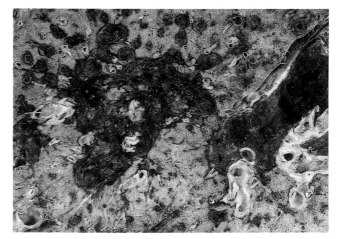

Fig.2.19 Coal workers' pneumoconiosis. The lung parenchyma shows patchy dense anthracotic pigmentation, a pattern known as dust reticulation. Note also the characteristic mild centrilobular 'focal dust' emphysema. In addition a small, black, silicotic nodule is present (arrowed). Simple dust reticulation results from long term exposure to coal dust; the development of nodules is due to co-inhalation of silica. There is *no* increased risk of lung cancer.

Fig.2.20 Progressive massive fibrosis. This coal miner's lung shows, in addition to dust reticulation, large, well demarcated, black fibrous masses and smaller black nodules (top). Progressive massive fibrosis affects up to 1% of coal miners and may also be seen in silicosis. The precise pathogenesis is unknown but it is thought that the degree of dust exposure and the possible coexistence of tuberculosis are important factors. The smaller nodules seen here are probably silicotic in nature, since coal dust often has a high silica content.

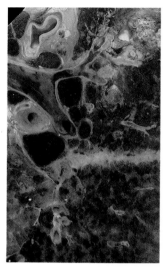

Fig.2.21 Silicosis. The lung parenchyma is markedly fibrotic, shows dense anthracotic pigmentation and contains a tuberculous cavity in the apex. The hilar nodes are black and enlarged and the interlobar fissure is scarred. Silicosis is seen most often in miners and workers in the stone and glass industries. Lung damage actually results from the release of macrophage cell contents following silica-induced cell death and is more usually characterised by nodular fibrosis (see Fig.2.22). Tuberculosis is a very common complication.

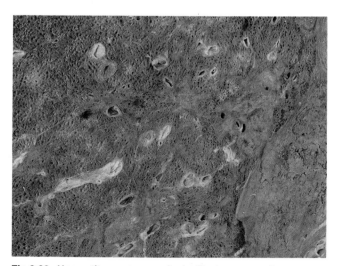

Fig.2.22 Haematite pneumoconiosis. The lung parenchyma shows severe brick-red pigmentation with evidence of nodular and diffuse fibrosis and emphysematous change. This condition, due to inhalation of iron oxide, is seen most often in iron ore miners. The development of fibrotic lesions is again dependent upon the co-existence of silica in the inhaled dust. Well recognised complications include tuberculosis and bronchial carcinoma.

CAUSES OF HONEYCOMB LUNG
Pneumoconiosis
Extrinsic allergic alveolitis
Cryptogenic fibrosing alveolitis (Hamman-Rich syndrome)
Sarcoidosis
Drugs/irradiation
Rheumatoid disease
Systemic sclerosis
Extensive pneumonia/TB
Pulmonary eosinophilia

Fig.2.23 Causes of honeycomb lung.

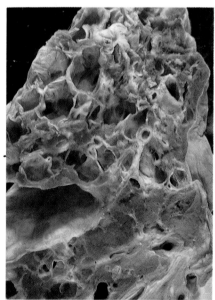

Fig.2.24 Honeycomb lung. The apex of the lung contains numerous variably-sized cystic spaces, each having a thick fibrous wall. These cysts represent gross dilatation of bronchioles and small bronchi in compensation for destruction and fibrosis of neighbouring alveoli and respiratory bronchioles. This appearance represents the end-stage of various disease processes, the commonest of which are listed in Fig. 2.23.

LUNG ACINUS

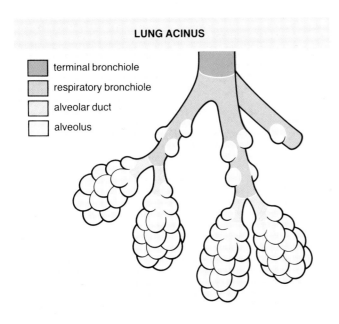

- terminal bronchiole
- respiratory bronchiole
- alveolar duct
- alveolus

Fig.2.25   A lung acinus. 3-5 pulmonary acini constitute a lung lobule.

CLASSIFICATION OF EMPHYSEMA
Centriacinar
Focal dust (in pneumoconiosis)
Panacinar
Paraseptal (bullous)
Irregular
Surgical (interstitial)

Fig.2.26   Classification of emphysema. With the exception of surgical emphysema, any lung may commonly show a mixed pattern of involvement.

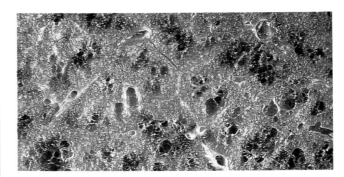

Fig.2.27   Centriacinar emphysema. In the lung parenchyma, small dilated air spaces surrounded by black anthracotic pigment are visible at the centre of the lung lobules. The surrounding alveoli are spared. These spaces correspond to the respiratory bronchioles and this is the commonest variant of emphysema, seen predominantly in cigarette smokers (especially males). The upper lobes, particularly the apices, are most often affected. A similar appearance is seen in coal workers (focal dust emphysema) in which there is usually little fibrosis or destruction.

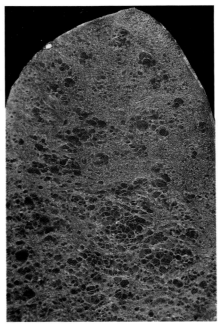

Fig.2.28   Panacinar emphysema. In this lung note the much larger, confluent, dilated air spaces replacing complete lung acini. In places there is also a centriacinar component. Panacinar emphysema, which is also very common, affects the air spaces, including alveoli, distal to the terminal bronchioles. In its classical form it is associated with α_1-antitrypsin deficiency and previous bronchial obstruction. Most often, the lower lobes, particularly the lung bases, are affected.

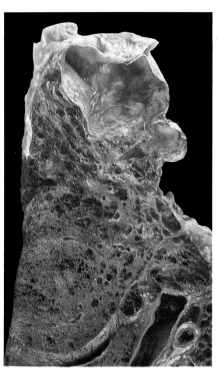

Fig.2.29 Paraseptal emphysema. At the apex of this lung is a large emphysematous bulla with a fibrous wall. The adjacent parenchyma shows mixed centri- and panacinar change. Paraseptal emphysema predominantly affects the alveoli adjacent to the interlobular septa or pleural surface. It is usually most pronounced in the upper lobes, often close to an area of previous scarring. This variant is the usual precursor of bullous emphysema and is often seen associated with other variants, as in this case.

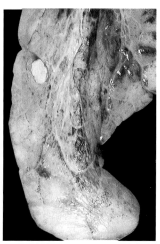

Fig.2.30 Pulmonary hamartoma. Just beneath the pleural surface of this lower lobe is a very well demarcated, small, pale tumour. The remainder of the lung is normal. Pulmonary hamartomas are not uncommon developmental anomalies, usually cartilaginous in nature, which are only rarely symptomatic. They are typically subpleural in location, affect males more than females, and are entirely benign.

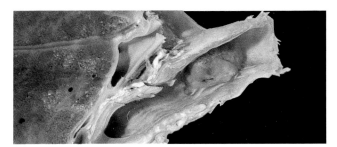

Fig.2.31 Bronchial 'adenoma'. In the main bronchus is a smooth, well circumscribed tumour projecting from the epithelial surface. These lesions may be derived either from submucosal glands or neuro endocrine APUD cells and are misnamed since they represent low-grade, malignant tumours which may eventually metastasise. They most often arise in young adults and there is usually extension into the adjacent lung parenchyma.

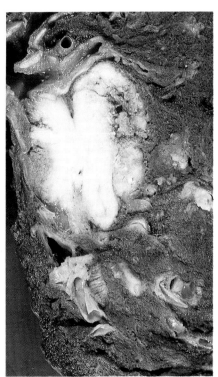

Fig.2.32 Hilar bronchial carcinoma. Arising from the lower lobe bronchus, close to the hilum, is a pale neoplasm which is irregularly infiltrating the parenchyma. Bronchial carcinoma most often originates near the hilum and may be squamous (50%), small cell (oat cell) anaplastic (20%), adeno-(15%) or large cell anaplastic (10%) in type. It is the commonest cause of death from malignancy in Great Britain and in many cases is associated with cigarette smoking or industrial exposure to carcinogens. The overall 5-year survival is only between 5 and 10%.

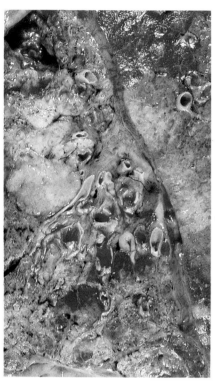

Fig.2.33 Bronchial carcinoma with distal bronchiectasis and bronchopneumonia. At the apex of the left lower lobe is a partly necrotic, pale neoplasm which has obliterated the lower lobe bronchus; distally the smaller bronchi are grossly dilated (bronchiectasis) and the remaining parenchyma shows consolidation. The adjacent middle lobe shows confluent bronchopneumonia. These are common complications of obstructive bronchial carcinoma and may also be accompanied by collapse or abscess formation.

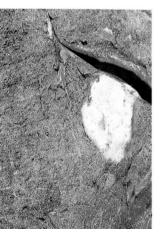

Fig.2.34 Peripheral lung carcinoma. Just beneath the pleura of the oblique interlobar fissure is an irregular, well demarcated, pale tumour which is situated well away from the main bronchial tree. The majority of peripheral primary pulmonary malignant tumours are adenocarcinomas which comprise about 10-15% of all lung cancers. These tumours show an equal sex incidence and tend to arise in foci of scarring. An apparently slow growth rate and frequent operability means that they carry a better prognosis than most bronchial carcinomas.

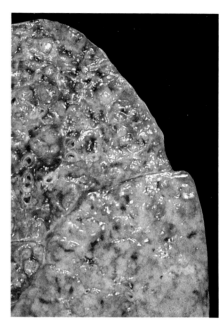

Fig.2.35 Bronchioalveolar carcinoma. The entire lung is diffusely infiltrated by a pale neoplasm which, particularly in the upper lobe, has adopted a nodular appearance. Bronchioalveolar carcinoma comprises about 2% of all primary lung cancers and is a specific variant of adenocarcinoma, which tends to spread extensively within the air passages. Its diffuse nature often prompts mistaken clinical diagnoses of an infective or interstitial disorder.

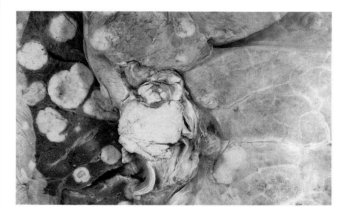

Fig.2.36 Multiple pulmonary metastases. Beneath the pleura and in the lung parenchyma are innumerable pale, umbilicated nodules of tumour. Up to a third of patients dying of malignant disease have pulmonary metastases, the commonest sources of which are carcinoma of the breast, colon, stomach and lung itself. The presence of an extensive vascular and lymphatic system in the lungs is responsible for the predilection that metastases show for this site.

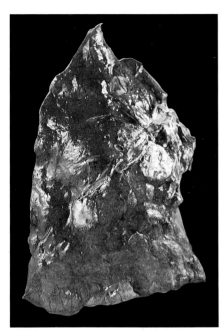

Fig.2.37 'Cannon ball' pulmonary metastases. In this congested lung, four well circumscribed, almost spherical, deposits of pale metastatic tumour are present. This appearance of a small number of large secondary deposits in the lung, while not entirely specific, is classically associated with spread from renal adenocarcinomas or testicular tumours.

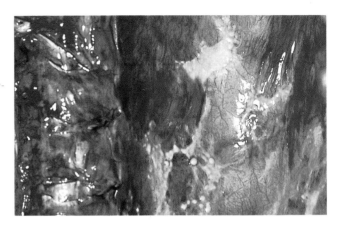

Fig.2.39 Pleural hyaline plaques. On the parietal pleura of the posterior thoracic wall are several foci of yellowish hyaline thickening. This appearance is most often seen in individuals who have suffered prolonged exposure to asbestos, usually in the course of their occupation. Such patients also commonly develop macroscopically non-specific pulmonary fibrosis, collapse or bronchiectasis of the lower lobes. Crocidolite is pathogenetically the most dangerous type of asbestos and occasionally only very brief exposure is sufficient to induce pulmonary disease.

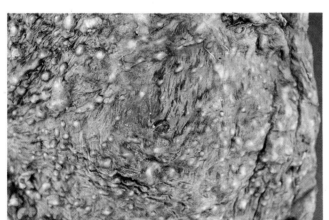

Fig.2.38 Pulmonary lymphangitis carcinomatosa. The pleural surface of this lung shows innumerable small spherical and linear deposits of pale tumour. This represents extensive infiltration of the pulmonary lymphatic channels, which are filled by neoplastic cells, and may be caused by either primary or secondary lung tumours.

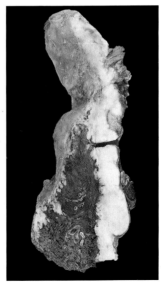

Fig.2.40 Mesothelioma. This apical portion of the lung is encased in pale, infiltrative tumour arising from the pleura. Involvement of the soft tissues at the apex is also apparent. Malignant mesothelioma is uncommon and may arise from the parietal or visceral pleura. The vast proportion of cases arise in patients exposed to asbestos, usually occupationally, and such individuals or their families are entitled to industrial compensation. The prognosis is uniformly appalling.

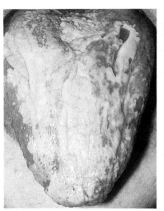

Fig. 3.1 Oral leukoplakia. This clinical photograph shows extensive smooth white patches over most of the tongue. Leukoplakia is purely a clinical description of any white plaque and is not a pathological diagnosis. In many cases, oral leukoplakia is benign, representing hyperkeratosis, the commonest causes of which are chronic irritation or smoking. Only cases which also show epithelial dysplasia can be regarded as premalignant. Other causes of white lesions in the oral cavity include lichen planus and candidiasis.

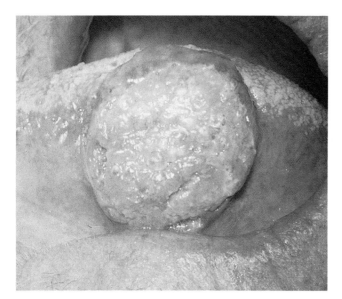

Fig. 3.2 Squamous carcinoma of tongue. This clinical photograph shows an irregular, raised pale lesion on the inferior surface of the patient's tongue. Most malignant tumours of the oral cavity are squamous carcinomas and postulated aetiological factors include tobacco smoking, syphilis and drinking strong spirits. They most commonly present in late adulthood, affecting predominantly males. The clinical course is very variable but carcinoma of the tongue generally carries a worse prognosis than tumours situated elsewhere in the mouth.

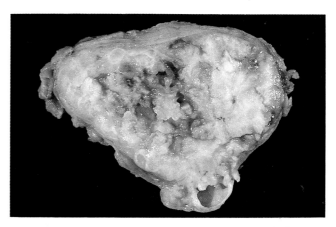

Fig. 3.3 Mixed salivary tumour (pleomorphic adenoma). This is the commonest neoplasm of salivary glands, the parotid being the most frequently affected site. This section shows a fairly well circumscribed, multinodular tumour; the cut surface has a myxoid cartilaginous appearance and there are small foci of cystic change and haemorrhage. These tumours are prone to local recurrence, most often as a consequence of spread through the capsule, which results in incomplete surgical excision. Malignant transformation is exceedingly rare.

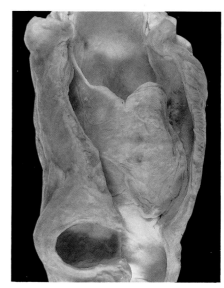

Fig. 3.4 Pharyngeal pouch. The pharynx has been opened posteriorly to show a diverticulum extending laterally. A pharyngeal pouch is a pulsion diverticulum which occurs at Killian's dehiscence, due to neuromuscular incoordination of the pharyngeal constrictor muscles. Elderly males are predominantly affected and very occasionally postcricoid carcinoma may develop in such a pouch.

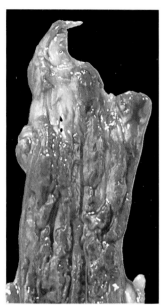

Fig. 3.5 Oesophageal candidiasis. Fungal infection of the oesophagus is not uncommon in immunocompromised patients, whether they be generally debilitated (particularly by malignant disease), receiving cytotoxic chemotherapy or suffering from a primary immunological disorder. The severity of the infection is dependent upon the degree of debility, and the appearance in the oesophagus may range from flat white plaques with minimal inflammation to greyish, ulcerated lesions with pseudomembrane formation and florid inflammation, as seen here.

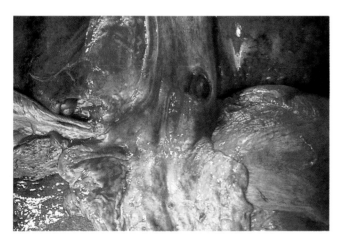

Fig. 3.6 Oesophagus - peptic (Barrett's) ulcer. A sharply demarcated ulcer with a haemorrhagic base is present in the lower third of the oesophagus. Barrett's ulcer occurs as a complication of either gastric metaplasia or heterotopia within the distal oesophagus. The commonest cause is chronic reflux oesophagitis, often in association with a hiatus hernia.

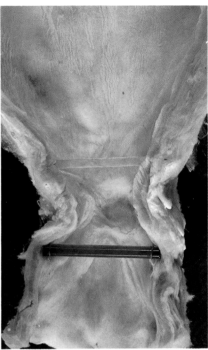

Fig. 3.7 Oesophageal stricture. The posterior aspect of the oesophagus has been displayed to show a zone of stricture formation complicated by the development of a small acute ulcer. Note the gross dilatation of the proximal (upper) oesophagus. Oesophageal strictures may be caused by a variety of conditions including reflux oesophagitis, peptic ulceration, ingestion of corrosives, scleroderma or trauma. Clearly, it is essential to distinguish such benign lesions from a stenosing carcinoma.

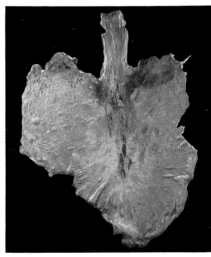

Fig. 3.8 Mallory-Weiss tear. The Mallory-Weiss syndrome is an uncommon cause of haematemesis, in which, most often, violent or prolonged vomiting results in tearing of the oesophageal or fundal mucosa with damage to the underlying blood vessels. It is particularly common in alcoholics.

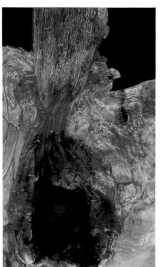

Fig.3.9 Oesophageal varices. These are dilated veins, situated predominantly in the lower oesophagus, which develop as a complication of chronic portal hypertension, most often due to cirrhosis of the liver. They are prone to rupture with resultant haematemesis. The oesophagus has been opened longitudinally to display numerous tortuous, dilated veins and, in the lower half of the picture, a mass of blood clot is present in the stomach.

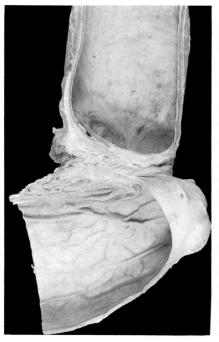

Fig. 3.10 Achalasia. The oesophagus and gastric fundus have been opened to display gross dilatation of the oesophageal lumen. The oesophago-gastric junction, not visible in this picture, was very narrow. In the posterior wall of the distal oesophagus are two pulsion diverticula. Achalasia is an idiopathic disorder of neuromuscular co-ordination affecting the autonomic plexus in the distal oesophagus; the oesophago-gastric junction fails to relax during swallowing resulting in proximal dilatation.

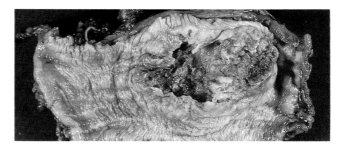

Fig.3.11 Carcinoma of the oesophagus. The oesophagus has been opened longitudinally to show an exophytic, largely ulcerated carcinoma in the middle third. Squamous carcinoma is the commonest malignant tumour of the oesophagus and most often affects older adults, predominantly males. Smoking and a high alcohol intake are thought to be causally related. Tumours in the upper third may rarely occur in association with the Plummer-Vinson syndrome which is almost exclusively seen in females. Tumours in the distal third of the oesophagus are most often adenocarcinomas which arise either in areas of gastric metaplasia or heterotopia, or represent infiltration by an adjacent gastric primary tumour.

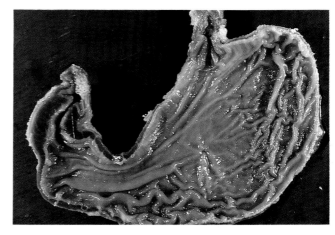

Fig. 3.12 Congenital pyloric stenosis. This infant's stomach has been opened to show marked hypertrophy of the muscle coat at the pylorus with obstruction and proximal dilatation. This condition is idiopathic but usually presents in the neonatal period with projectile vomiting. It occurs in approximately 1 in 500 live births, is commonly familial and affects males more than females. The mode of inheritance appears to be multifactorial. If untreated, the patient may develop profound metabolic alkalosis.

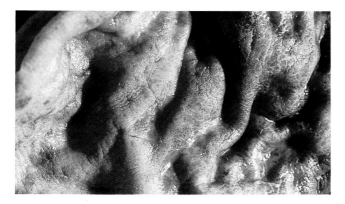

Fig. 3.13 Acute gastritis. This stomach has been opened to show a normal rugal pattern with marked mucosal congestion on the right hand side (cf. the pyloric antrum on the left). Acute gastritis is defined as transient mucosal inflammation, the commonest causes of which are salicylates, excess alcohol intake, cytotoxic drugs or hypotensive shock (of whatever cause). Added intramucosal oedema and haemorrhage may lead to the development of small mucosal erosions.

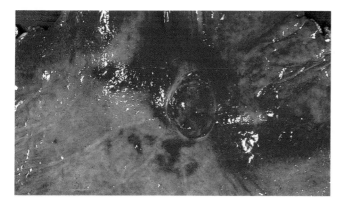

Fig.3.14 Acute gastric ulcer. The stomach has been opened to show a shallow, punched-out haemorrhagic ulcer with smooth edges. Acute peptic ulcers represent an extension of acute gastritis or gastric erosions and as such have largely the same causes. They may be differentiated from an erosion by their involvement of the submucosa as well as the mucosa. Acute ulcers rarely exceed 1cm in diameter. Less common associated causes include severe burns (Curling's ulcer) or cerebral injury and neurosurgery (Cushing's ulcer).

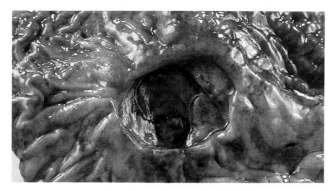

Fig. 3.15 Chronic gastric (peptic) ulcer. The stomach has been opened to show a sharply demarcated ulcer with straight edges, which has penetrated the muscular layer of the gastric wall; its base is composed of smooth but irregularly heaped-up granulation and scar tissue. Chronic gastric ulcers affect males more than females, usually in middle life and are more common in patients with blood group O. Most patients are usually hypochlorhydric and it is thought that relative mucosal ischaemia, an impaired mucosal mucous barrier, altered gastric emptying rate or reflux of bile acids from the duodenum may be important pathogenetic factors. These ulcers are usually solitary and the vast proportion arise at the border zone between acid-secreting and non-acid-secreting mucosa, particularly on the lesser curve.

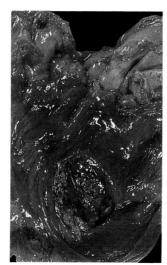

Fig.3.16 Bleeding gastric ulcer. Chronic peptic ulcers commonly damage small arteries or veins as they erode the stomach wall. Haemorrhage is therefore the most frequent complication: this may either occur in small amounts over a long period of time, resulting in melaena and iron-deficiency anaemia, or a larger vessel may bleed acutely and heavily, giving rise to haematemesis. There is clotted blood in the floor of this ulcer and blood in the stomach. Note also the smaller peptic ulcer just above the main lesion.

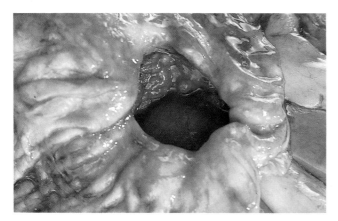

Fig. 3.17 Perforated gastric ulcer. Perforation of chronic peptic ulcers, i.e. disruption of the full thickness of the stomach wall, occurs in up to 5% of cases. This is a life-threatening complication which results in peritonitis. In this specimen, while a small area of granulation tissue remains at the superior border of the ulcer, perforation has occurred and part of the left lobe of the liver is visible through the floor of the lesion.

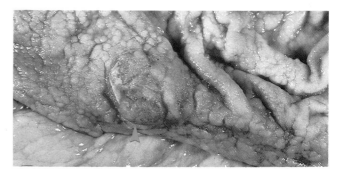

Fig.3.19 Gastric adenoma. At the edge of the greater curve is a small, rounded, raised lesion projecting from the mucosal surface (arrowed). There is no evidence of ulceration or adjacent infiltration. Gastric adenomas, more accurately known as neoplastic polyps, may be classified like those in the large bowel (see Figs.3.45 and 3.46) although they are only rarely pedunculated. They have exactly the same malignant potential and are often seen in association with chronic atrophic gastritis.

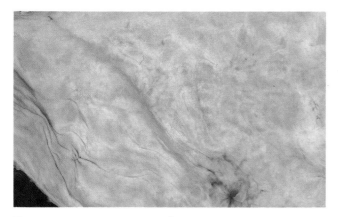

Fig. 3.18 Chronic atrophic gastritis. This stomach shows extreme atrophy and pallor with loss of the mucosal folds and marked attenuation of the gastric wall, such that it is almost translucent. This represents the end-stage of chronic autoimmune gastritis, which is the commonest cause of pernicious anaemia. Autoantibodies to intrinsic factor and gastric parietal cells are found in such patients, who develop a marked deficiency of vitamin B_{12}. Up to 10% of patients with atrophic gastritis may subsequently develop gastric carcinoma.

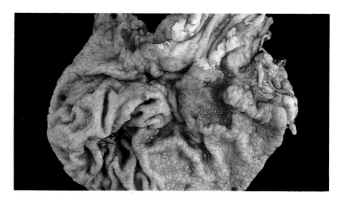

Fig. 3.20 Gastric adenocarcinoma. In the fundus of the stomach is an ulcerated neoplasm with irregular rolled edges. Adenocarcinoma of the stomach is one of the most common causes of death due to malignancy in Britain, occurring most often in elderly men. There is a familial incidence and patients with blood group A are at increased risk. Geographically, the disease is most common in Japan and Scandinavia. Currently favoured aetiological agents are nitrosamines, derived from ingested nitrates which are used in preservatives and crop fertilisers. Known predisposing conditions include chronic atrophic gastritis and uncommonly, gastric adenomata. Macroscopically, ulcerating tumours are far more common than the fungating or polypoid forms.

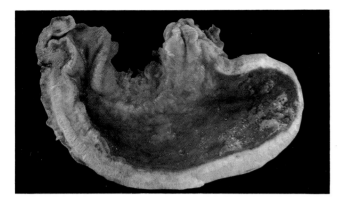

Fig. 3.21 Linitis plastica ('leather-bottle' stomach). The stomach has been dissected to show diffuse infiltration of much of the greater curve by pale, rigid tumour, resulting in shrinkage of the gastric lumen. This macroscopic variant of adenocarcinoma of the stomach represents widespread infiltration by poorly differentiated tumour with an associated dense fibrous (desmoplastic) stroma. Since these tumours only rarely impinge on the gastric lumen, they commonly present at an advanced stage and the prognosis is very poor.

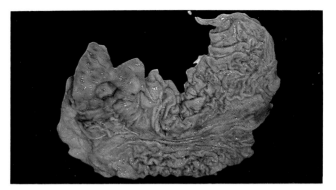

Fig. 3.23 Chronic duodenal ulcer. The stomach and proximal duodenum have been opened to show a well circumscribed, deep ulcer with smooth edges in the first part of the duodenum. Duodenal peptic ulcers are much commoner than their gastric counterparts and are seen most frequently in males between the ages of 20 and 40. In contrast to gastric ulcers, these lesions are associated with marked hyperacidity, the precise cause of which is uncertain. They occur most often in the first part, particularly on the anterior wall and produce similar complications to ulcers in the stomach.

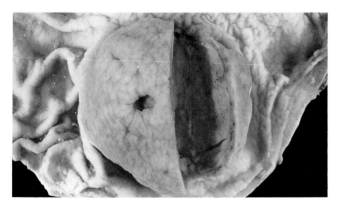

Fig. 3.22 Gastric leiomyoma. The stomach has been opened to show a smooth, rounded and well circumscribed tumour, with a small ulcer at its apex. The cut surface (right) reveals that the tumour is covered by a layer of attenuated, normal epithelium. Leiomyomas are not uncommon benign gastric tumours, which are often asymptomatic. They arise within the muscular coat of the stomach and, when projecting into the gastric lumen, are very prone to superficial ulceration. Their malignant counterpart, leiomyosarcoma, is extremely rare.

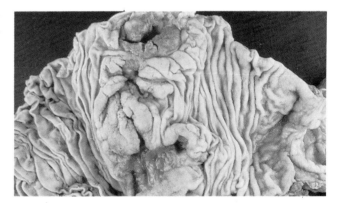

Fig. 3.24 Periampullary carcinoma. This segment of duodenum has been opened to show a fungating, focally ulcerated tumour arising around the ampulla of Vater. The pyloric canal is apparent on the right. Periampullary carcinoma arises from the distal end of the common bile duct and occurs most often in older adults. It is usually slow-growing and carries a relatively good prognosis. It is very important to distinguish such cases from carcinoma of the head of the pancreas, which presents very similarly, since surgical intervention is undoubtedly worthwhile in periampullary tumours.

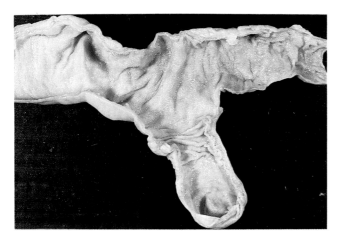

Fig.3.25 Meckel's diverticulum. This opened segment of ileum shows a wide diverticulum, about 2 cm in diameter, lined by rather smooth mucosa. Meckel's diverticulum is a congenital malformation representing a remnant of the vitello-intestinal duct. Usually found about 60 cm from the ileocaecal valve, it affects about 2% of the population. While it may become inflamed or obstructed, ectopic gastric mucosa is present in some cases, which may lead to peptic ulceration. Other ectopic epithelia which are often found include pancreatic, duodenal and colonic types.

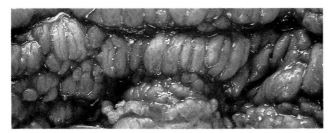

Fig. 3.26 Crohn's disease. This opened length of small bowel shows the typical 'cobblestone' appearance of the mucosa, each nodule being separated by ulcerated fissures. Crohn's disease is an idiopathic granulomatous condition which may affect any site in the alimentary tract but shows a predilection for the terminal ileum. It presents most often in the 2nd to 4th decades. Postulated aetiological agents include various micro-organisms and fine particulate matter, which have induced an abnormal immunological response. Multifocal involvement, giving rise to 'skip' lesions, is characteristic and inflammation of the full thickness of the bowel wall causes deep fissuring, fistula formation and fibrosis.

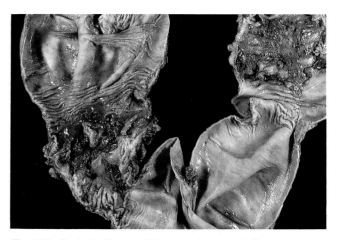

Fig. 3.27 Crohn's disease. This opened segment of large bowel shows two quite separate 'skip' lesions, characterised by florid mucosal ulceration. The lesion on the left has induced marked luminal stenosis with obvious proximal dilatation. Up to 15% of patients with Crohn's disease show large bowel involvement, with or without small intestinal disease. There is a definite increased risk of colonic adenocarcinoma, but this is much less marked than in ulcerative colitis.

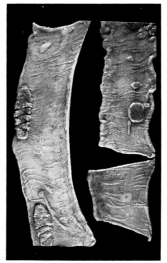

Fig. 3.28 Typhoid ulceration. These segments of small intestine have been opened to show several ovoid ulcers lying parallel to the bowel wall (cf. Fig. 3.29). The ulceration has occurred at the site of necrosis of Peyer's patches. Typhoid fever remains endemic in some parts of the world, especially Asia and the Far East. It is due to ingestion of food or drink contaminated with *Salmonella typhi*, usually from an asymptomatic carrier. Important local complications include perforation and haemorrhage. Following invasion of the bloodstream, excretion of *Salmonellae* in bile may lead to chronic gallbladder infection (whence the carrier state).

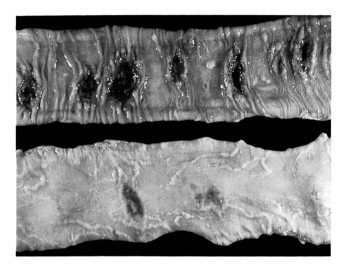

Fig. 3.29 Intestinal tuberculosis. In contrast to Fig. 3.28, this ulceration, while still originating in Peyer's patches, extends transversely around the bowel wall following the lines of lymphatic drainage. Intestinal tuberculosis may be primary, resulting from ingestion of unpasteurised milk, or secondary, as a consequence of swallowing infected sputum from pulmonary disease. Adjacent lymph nodes are usually involved and may later undergo dystrophic calcification. Peritoneal involvement may lead to ascites.

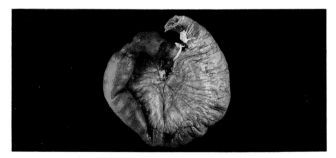

Fig. 3.30 Small intestinal ischaemia. This loop of bowel is dilated and markedly congested. This is the appearance of infarction of the bowel wall, but lesser degrees of ischaemia may result only in mucosal ulceration. It most commonly results from an embolus, usually cardiac in origin, occluding a branch of the superior mesenteric artery. Other causes include severe hypotension, thrombosis in an atheromatous vessel, retrograde infarction due to mesenteric venous thrombosis or digitalis therapy.

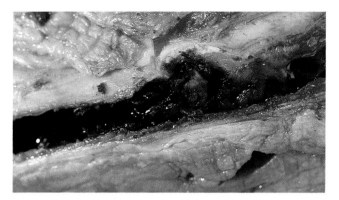

Fig. 3.31 Mesenteric embolism. The superior mesenteric artery is totally occluded by thrombus which has embolised from the left atrium in this patient with atrial fibrillation. Proximal occlusion, such as this, results in infarction of almost the entire small bowel and is invariably fatal.

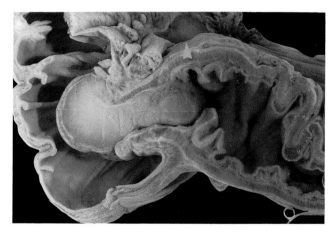

Fig.3.32 Carcinoid tumour. The terminal ileum and caecum are shown here. Originating in the ileocaecal valve is a well circumscribed, yellow tumour in the submucosa. In the adjacent mesenteric fat, a lymph node containing metastatic tumour can be seen (arrowed). Carcinoid tumours arise from neuroendocrine APUD cells and are usually found in the appendix or small intestine. Tumours in the appendix tend to be solitary and affect young adults, while those in the small bowel may be multiple and usually present in old people. The appendiceal neoplasms almost never metastasise, but small bowel tumours frequently spread to lymph nodes and the liver.

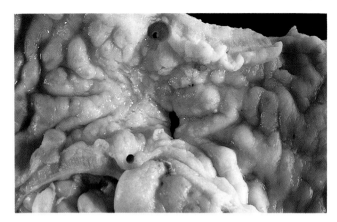

Fig. 3.33 Intestinal lymphoma. This segment of bowel shows a solitary, ulcerated tumour. Macroscopically, primary gastro-intestinal lymphoma may be indistinguishable from a carcinoma. Involvement by disseminated lymphoma usually gives rise to multiple lesions and may therefore be more easily recognised. Gastro-intestinal lymphomas are nearly all non-Hodgkin's in type. There is an increased incidence associated with coeliac disease and α heavy chain disease.

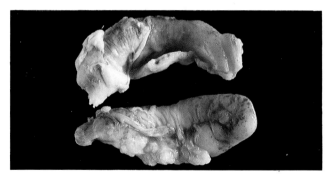

Fig. 3.34 Acute appendicitis. The appendix below shows marked serosal congestion while the one above is covered in a fibrino-purulent exudate, indicative of more advanced infection. The aetio-logy of acute appendicitis is still debated but it is thought that luminal obstruction, usually by faecal material, probably leads to mucosal ulceration followed by penetration of the bowel wall by a variety of faecal organisms. Occasional fatalities still occur in elderly or very young patients who develop perforation and peritonitis. Other com-plications include the development of an empyema or mucocoele of the appendix.

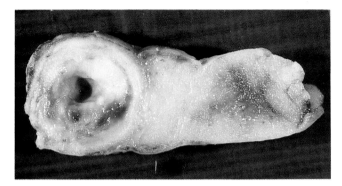

Fig. 3.35 Acute appendicitis. This appendix has been sectioned transversely to show copious intraluminal and intramural purulent material associated with congestion and haemorrhage in the wall and adjacent mesenteric fat.

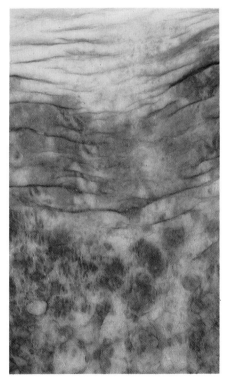

Fig. 3.36 Ulcerative colitis. The distal portion of this rectum has a granular, almost velvety, appearance with haemorrhage and innumerable shallow ulcers. The proximal margin (above) appears normal. Ulcerative colitis is an idio-pathic disease, pre-dominantly of young adults, which always involves the rectum and affects the proximal large bowel in continuity. It is a chronic relapsing condition primarily affecting the mucosa. It is assoc-iated with HLA B-27 and may be com-plicated by toxic megacolon, per-foration and the development of adenocarcinoma.

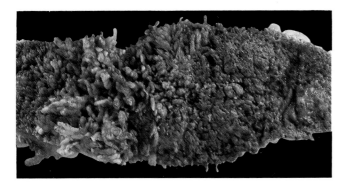

Fig. 3.37 Pseudo-polyps in ulcerative colitis. This segment of large bowel shows intense mucosal congestion and, in addition, the mucosa is 'thrown up' into innumerable irregular polypoid protrusions. These are not true polyps but simply represent the effects of adjacent ulceration, undermining the mucosa with granulation tissue formation. Even when the disease is in remission, these tags may persist as elevated areas between the healed atrophic foci of previously ulcerated mucosa.

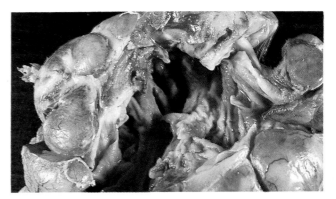

Fig. 3.39 Diverticulitis. This sigmoid colon has been opened to show mucosal congestion associated with a florid, serosal, fibrino-purulent exudate. In the lumen, the ostia of several diverticula are visible. Inflammation complicating diverticular disease results from mucosal ulceration due to inspissation of faecal material within diverticula. Diverticulitis can be either acute or chronic and may give rise to fibrosis or perforation.

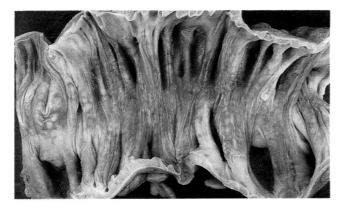

Fig. 3.38 Diverticular disease. This sigmoid colon has been opened to show two almost parallel rows of diverticular ostia. In the Western World, diverticular disease of the colon is extremely common, particularly with advancing age. It results from the effects of increased intraluminal pressure consequent upon the peristaltic contractions required to propel the more viscid or solid faecal material, characteristic of a diet low in fibre. The condition may be complicated by attacks of acute or chronic inflammation, perforation or haemorrhage. Diverticular disease *does not* predispose to colonic adenocarcinoma.

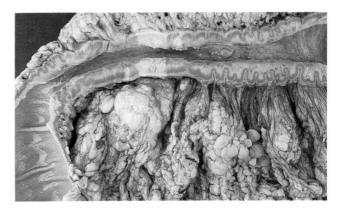

Fig. 3.40 Chronic ischaemic colitis. This large bowel has been opened from behind to show an area of mucosal congestion associated with fibrous thickening of the bowel wall and stricture formation. The appearance is typical of long-standing relative ischaemia which usually results from mesenteric arterial disease without complete occlusion (cf. Fig.3.30). Commonly, ischaemic colitis is complicated by bacterial infection and progressive fibrosis: as a consequence, the macroscopical appearances can be confused with those of inflammatory bowel disease or malignancy.

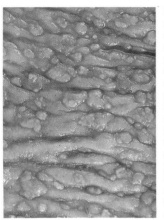

Fig. 3.41 Pseudo-membranous colitis. This close-up view of large bowel mucosa shows numerous small, raised, yellowish plaques. The appearance is virtually diagnostic of pseudomembranous colitis and is usually found in the left side of the colon. The condition occurs most often following a course of antibiotics, which, in altering the natural flora and susceptibility of the colon to bacterial colonisation, allows infection with *Clostridium difficile* (a Gram-positive anaerobe) and the elaboration of its potent exotoxin to occur.

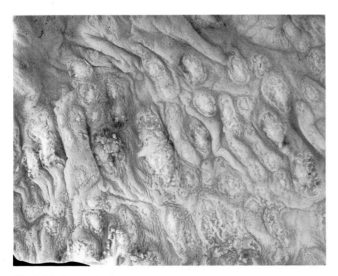

Fig. 3.42 Amoebic dysentery. The colon shows irregular foci of mucosal congestion and swelling with adjacent areas of ulceration. Amoebic dysentery results from infection with the protozoon *Entamoeba histolytica*, which is endemic in the tropics. After ingestion, the organisms invade the bowel wall and cause submucosal necrosis, which results in 'flask-shaped' ulcers with sparing of the overlying mucosa in the early stages. Complications include chronic infection, with fibrosis or exuberant formation of granulation tissue (the 'amoeboma'), and infection of the portal venous system (see Fig.4.4).

CLASSIFICATION OF LARGE BOWEL POLYPS		
Anomalous mucosal fold		
'Metaplastic' (hyperplastic)		
Inflammatory pseudo-polyp		
Lymphoid		
Hamartomatous	juvenile	
	Peutz-Jeghers	
Neoplastic (adenoma)	tubular	
	tubulo-villous	
	villous	

Fig. 3.43 Classification of large bowel polyps.

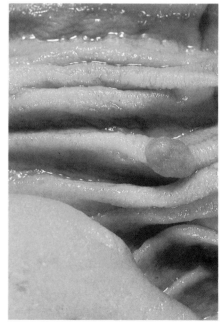

Fig. 3.44 'Metaplastic' polyp. This close-up view of large bowel mucosa shows a very small, pale, polypoid nodule situated on the crest of one of the mucosal folds. 'Metaplastic' polyps are, in fact, hyperplastic lesions showing an increased cell turnover. They occur in the large bowel and may be found at any age, but are especially common from the 5th decade onwards. They are usually multiple, small, flat or sessile and arise most often in the rectum. They have no malignant potential.

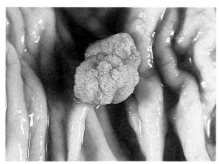

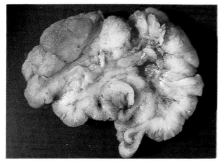

Fig.3.45 Tubular adenoma. A typical example of a tubular adenoma projecting from the mucosa of the large bowel (upper). A separate specimen (lower) has been bisected to show its smooth, lobulated appearance and small pedicle. Neoplastic polyps of the large bowel are very common in Western society, particularly with increasing age. This most frequent variant of a neoplastic polyp is usually less than 3cm in diameter. They are often multiple and are all pre-malignant.

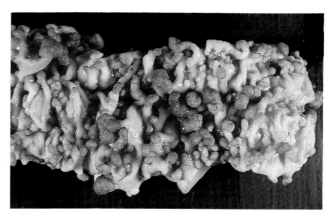

Fig. 3.47 Familial polyposis coli. This segment of large bowel is covered in numerous tubular adenomas of varying size. Polyposis coli is a rare autosomal dominant inherited condition in which patients develop hundreds of large bowel adenomas, usually in the 2nd and 3rd decades. Close screening of all family members is obligatory since, if these patients are left untreated, all will develop one or more adenocarcinomas over a period of 10-20 years. Despite such efforts, up to 40% of cases have a colonic carcinoma at presentation.

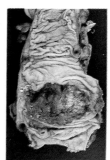 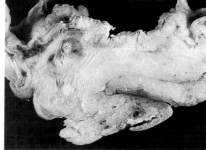

Fig. 3.48 Ulcerating rectal carcinoma. The distal end of this opened rectum (left) shows an ulcerated tumour with irregular rolled edges. A similar tumour (right) has been sectioned to show penetration of the muscle coat and a lymph node containing metastatic tumour is visible in the mesenteric fat. Adenocarcinoma of the large bowel is the second commonest cause of death from malignancy in Britain, even though up to 45% of patients are cured. It arises most often in the left side of the bowel. There is a familial tendency and postulated aetiological factors include a low fibre diet, a high fat diet and a dietary alteration in bile salt metabolism. Prognosis is directly related to staging (see Fig. 3.52).

Fig. 3.46 Villous adenoma. This example has been photographed *en face* to show that it is a large, broad-based sessile lesion from which numerous irregular papillary fronds project. Note that the margins of this polyp are ill-defined. This variant of neoplastic polyp is most common in the rectum. It tends to be larger and show more severe dysplasia than the tubular adenoma and, as such, more commonly progresses to adenocarcinoma. Villous adenomas of the rectum may sometimes secrete large amounts of potassium or albumin, giving rise to symptoms of hypokalaemia or hypoalbuminaemia.

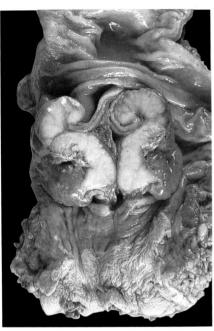

Fig. 3.49 Fungating rectal carcinoma. This is an abdomino-perineal resection specimen showing a 'cauliflower' fungating tumour, in the distal rectum, which has been bisected to emphasise its polypoid mode of growth. This macroscopical variant of large bowel adenocarcinoma is comparatively uncommon and is usually histologically well differentiated.

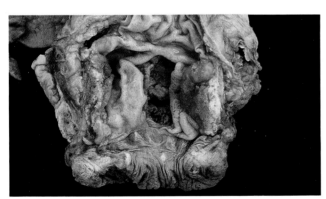

Fig. 3.50 Annular stenosing rectal carcinoma. This is another abdomino-perineal resection specimen. The tumour can be seen to encircle the entire lumen of the bowel and shows central ulceration. Circumferential spread may be facilitated by extension of the tumour through submucosal lymphatics. This macroscopical variant is particularly likely to give rise to large bowel obstruction with proximal dilatation, stercoral ulceration and possible perforation.

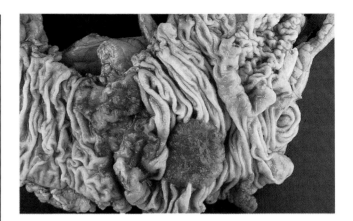

Fig. 3.51 Caecal carcinoma. The terminal ileum and caecum have been dissected to show three separate lesions arising in the proximal caecal mucosa. The largest (left) is an ulcerated adenocarcinoma while the other two are neoplastic polyps. Adenocarcinoma of the caecum is commoner in females and, owing to the distensibility of the caecum, gives rise to symptoms less often. Insidious blood loss, possibly with melaena, may lead to presentation as iron-deficiency anaemia. This specimen demonstrates the frequency with which neoplastic polyps and carcinoma are found in the same specimen.

DUKES' STAGING OF COLORECTAL ADENOCARCINOMA

Stage	A	B	C
Extent of tumour	Confined to bowel wall	Invasion through bowel wall	Lymph node metastases
5 - year survival	90%	65%	20%
mucosa muscularis mucosae muscularis propria serosa fat lymph nodes			

Fig.3.52 Dukes' staging, conceived by Cuthbert Dukes, St. Mark's Hospital, London.

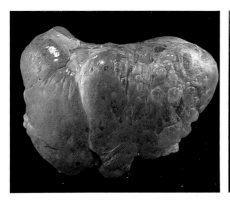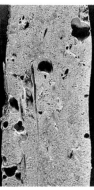

Fig.4.1 Polycystic liver. The anterior surface of the liver (left) shows numerous, multiloculated subcapsular cysts, predominantly in the left lobe. On the right, a separate case shows the cut-surface appearance. Polycystic disease of the liver is an inherited autosomal dominant condition, frequently associated with adult polycystic renal disease. In general it does not impair liver function. A similar, though usually less marked, appearance may be seen in congenital hepatic fibrosis.

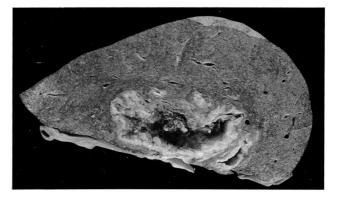

Fig.4.3 Hepatic abscess. Within the liver parenchyma is a large abscess cavity, lined by purulent material, and showing central necrosis. There is also an adjacent smaller lesion. Hepatic abscesses most often complicate suppurative cholangitis or portal pyaemia, as may be seen in diverticulitis or appendicitis. Such abscesses are commonly multiple and are usually due to infection by gut flora such as Gram-negative or anaerobic bacteria.

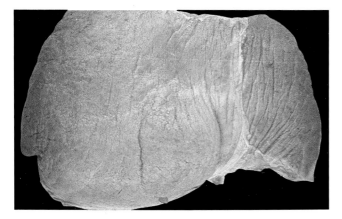

Fig.4.2 Massive hepatic necrosis. The liver is pink and mildly shrunken; the capsule has a wrinkled, rather loose appearance. Massive hepatic necrosis is uncommon but is most frequently associated with fulminant viral hepatitis (usually hepatitis B or non-A non-B); it may also be caused by other hepatotoxic agents including such drugs as halothane, methyldopa and isoniazid. The prognosis is generally poor and acute hepatic failure rapidly supervenes.

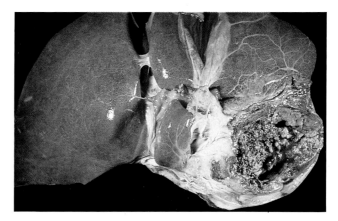

Fig.4.4 Hepatic amoebic 'abscess'. In the posterior aspect of the right lobe is a large necrotic cavity showing surrounding fibrosis. The contents of the cavity are said to bear some resemblance to anchovy sauce. Hepatic involvement by *Entamoeba histolytica* occurs via the portal venous system (see Fig.3.42) and may be seen in up to 30% of cases of amoebiasis. Necrosis, as seen here, is caused by the protozoa and is the commonest manifestation but it should be noted that no true suppuration occurs.

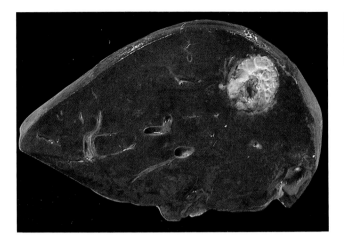

Fig.4.5 Hepatic hydatid cyst. A transverse section through this liver shows a well circumscribed loculated fibrous cyst. Hydatid disease is due to infestation by the tapeworm *Echinococcus granulosus*, and is seen most often in sheep-farming communities. Spread to the liver occurs via the portal system from the duodenum and affects at least 50% of cases. Such cysts are usually solitary, are found most often in the right lobe and contain many daughter cysts with brood capsules and scolices. The case here appears to be 'burnt-out'.

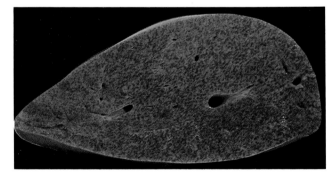

Fig.4.6 Passive hepatic venous congestion. The cut surface of the liver has a variegated appearance, reminiscent of a nutmeg, with small multifocal areas of congestion surrounded by a rim of pale tissue. This appearance is the result of chronic congestive cardiac failure with centrilobular venous congestion and atrophy, or occasionally fatty change, of the adjacent parenchyma. In some cases there may be associated fibrosis, but the development of true cirrhosis is an extremely rare complication.

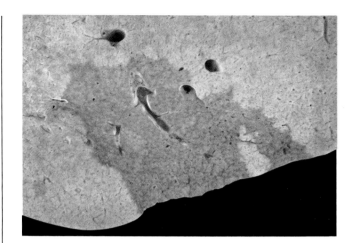

Fig.4.7 Hepatic Zahn infarct. In this close-up view, an approximately wedge-shaped area of subcapsular parenchyma shows a congested pseudo-infarct with slight concavity of the overlying capsule. This is the typical appearance which results from thrombosis of a portal vein radicle, usually as a consequence of a small embolus or compression by tumour. The hepatic arterial supply prevents true infarction in such cases, but parenchymal atrophy and sinusoidal congestion occur.

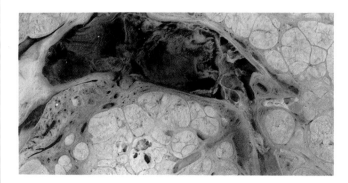

Fig.4.8 Portal vein thrombosis. A large branch of the portal vein is totally occluded by thrombus. Note that the liver parenchyma shows florid macronodular cirrhosis. Portal vein thrombosis is most often associated with either local venous obstruction by a neoplasm, intra-abdominal sepsis or recent abdominal surgery. While passive splenic congestion commonly ensues, true hepatic infarction does not occur unless the blood supply from the hepatic artery is also compromised.

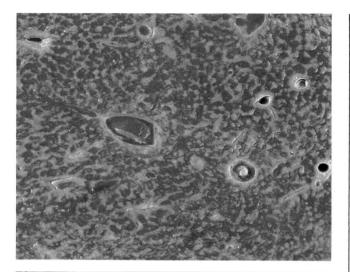

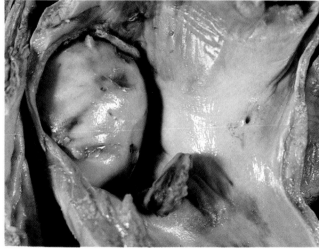

Fig.4.9 Budd-Chiari syndrome. The liver parenchyma (top) shows an exaggerated 'nutmeg' pattern (see Fig.4.6) and several tributaries of the hepatic vein are occluded by thrombus. A mass of tumour (bottom) occupies the lumen of the inferior vena cava. This was a primary leiomyosarcoma. This rare syndrome is due to thrombosis of the principal hepatic veins or inferior vena cava, and may be due to endophlebitis, obstruction by tumour either primary (as in this case), secondary or adjacent, or associated with polycythaemia rubra vera.

CAUSES OF HEPATIC FATTY CHANGE
Alcohol abuse
Starvation/malnutrition
Diabetes mellitus
Glycogen storage diseases
Galactosaemia
Pregnancy   acute idiopathic fatty change   fatty change with hyperemesis
Severe systemic infection
Pathological obesity
Cystic fibrosis
Drugs, especially tetracycline
Chemical toxins, such as carbon tetrachloride
Reye's syndrome

Fig.4.10 Causes of hepatic fatty change.

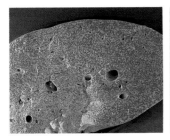 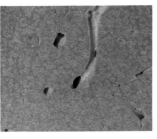

Fig.4.11 Hepatic fatty change. On the left, the liver parenchyma is diffusely yellowish and, on the right, a portion of a similar liver has been stained with Scharlach R which stains the fat orange-red. Fatty change represents excessive cytoplasmic accumulation of neutral lipid and triglyceride and, as a consequence of its important metabolic role, the liver is particularly liable to be affected. Alcohol abuse is the commonest cause in the Western World but, on a global scale, malnutrition is probably the single most important factor.

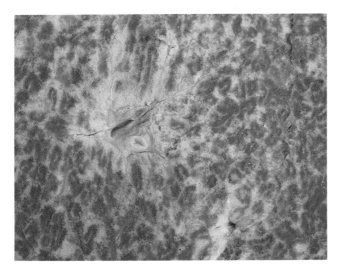

Fig.4.12 Hepatic amyloid deposition. The liver parenchyma, originally rather waxy in appearance, has been stained with Congo Red to show extensive deposition of amyloid, particularly in the mid-zone of the lobules. Hepatic amyloidosis is most often secondary in type, being composed of serum amyloid A protein. Common causes of secondary amyloidosis include chronic infection or chronic inflammatory disorders such as rheumatoid arthritis. While the liver may become enlarged and firm, functional impairment is rare despite a degree of parenchymal atrophy.

CAUSES OF CIRRHOSIS
Alcohol abuse
Post-viral (hepatitis B/non-A, non-B/δ agent)
Biliary (primary or secondary)
Haemochromatosis
Wilson's disease
α_1 - antitrypsin deficiency
Indian childhood
Metabolic storage disorders
Drugs (methyldopa, isoniazid)

Fig.4.13 Causes of cirrhosis. 10-15% of cases remain idiopathic.

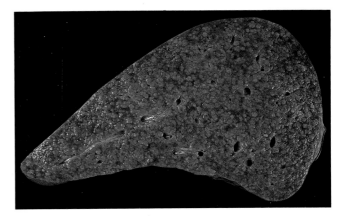

Fig.4.14 Micronodular cirrhosis. The liver is small and the cut surface shows multiple small, pale nodules which are rather uniform in appearance. Micronodular cirrhosis (nodules < 3mm in diameter) is classically seen in alcohol abuse and haemochromatosis. Worldwide, alcohol is by far the most common cause of cirrhosis and the incidence is increasing. Complications include portal hypertension, splenomegaly, ascites, encephalopathy and clotting abnormalities.

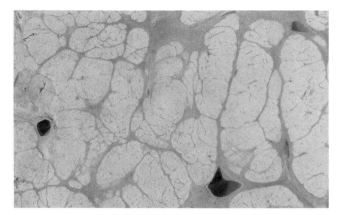

Fig.4.15 Macronodular cirrhosis. This close-up view shows the cut surface of the liver to be composed of large (>3mm), pale nodules of varying size, each separated by dense fibrous bands. Typically, a macronodular pattern is a feature of post-viral (usually Hepatitis B) cirrhosis and Wilson's disease. Note, however, that many cirrhotic livers show a mixed pattern, irrespective of aetiology.

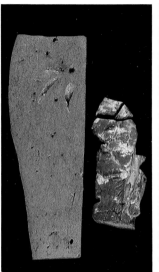

Fig.4.17 Haemochromatosis. The pancreas (right) and, to a lesser extent, the cut surface of the liver show deep brown pigmentation, due largely to excessive deposition of haemosiderin. Idiopathic haemochromatosis is an autosomal dominantly-inherited condition, characterised by defective iron metabolism, which results in massive iron deposition, particularly in the liver, pancreas, heart, adrenals and skin. Males are most often affected and typically present in middle age. Complications include the development of cirrhosis, hepatocellular carcinoma, diabetes mellitus, cardiac failure and Addison's disease.

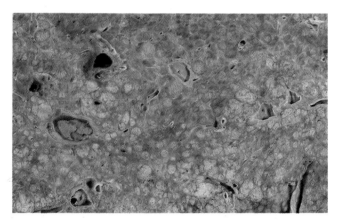

Fig.4.16 Biliary cirrhosis. The cut surface of this liver shows a micronodular pattern, associated with marked green bile-staining. Biliary cirrhosis, which is uncommon, is most often primary in type. This is an idiopathic condition which usually affects middle-aged females, is associated with anti-mitochondrial antibodies and may be autoimmune in origin. Very rarely, a similar appearance may be seen secondary to long-standing, extra-hepatic obstruction or mucoviscidosis.

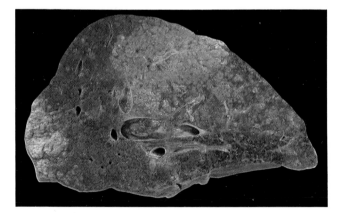

Fig.4.18 Hepatoma with micronodular cirrhosis. The liver is diffusely nodular but, in addition, two irregular areas of pale, neoplastic tissue are apparent. The larger, central portion of tumour has invaded the main hepatic vein. Hepatoma, (primary hepatocellular carcinoma) is not uncommon and is seen most often in Africa and the Far East. A high proportion of cases are associated with pre-existent cirrhosis, particularly alcoholic, viral and that associated with haemochromatosis. Other known causes include aflatoxins (from mouldy grain) and various alkaloids e.g. from herbal teas.

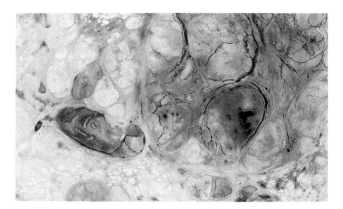

Fig.4.19　Multinodular hepatoma. The liver parenchyma is diffusely replaced by numerous greenish nodules of tumour. Between these nodules, the uninvolved hepatic tissue shows a micronodular cirrhosis. It is unknown whether this pattern of hepatocellular carcinoma represents multifocality of origin or intrahepatic metastasis. Occasionally hepatomas may display a diffuse micronodular infiltrative appearance which may be difficult to distinguish macroscopically from cirrhosis. The aetiological factors and prognosis of hepatoma are identical, irrespective of the gross appearance.

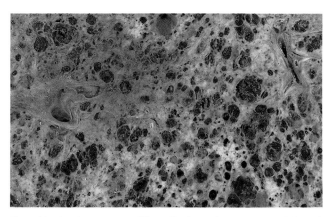

Fig.4.20　Angiosarcoma of liver. The hepatic parenchyma is largely replaced by a diffuse haemorrhagic neoplasm in which multiple small vascular channels are visible. Hepatic angiosarcoma is rare and may arise either in infants or, more usually, in adults. Adult cases may be associated with previous exposure to the contrast medium, Thorotrast, or to vinyl chloride monomer in the plastics industry. In general the prognosis is extremely poor.

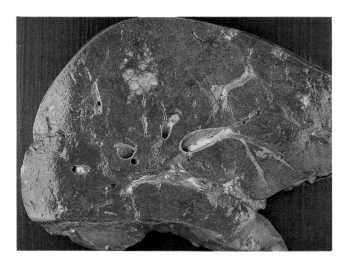

Fig.4.21　Hepatic metastases. Multiple irregular nodules of pale secondary tumour are randomly distributed in the parenchyma of this otherwise normal liver. Metastatic involvement of the liver is extremely common and occurs most often in association with primary tumours drained by the portal venous system, particularly gastro-intestinal adenocarcinomas. The liver is also a very common site of secondary spread from carcinomas of the bronchus and breast and malignant melanoma. Metastases are very uncommon in cirrhotic livers, probably as a consequence of alterations in hepatic blood flow.

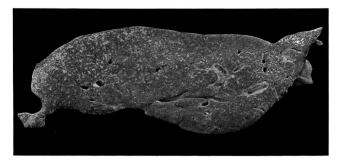

Fig.4.22　Hepatic involvement by lymphoma. Throughout the liver parenchyma there is diffuse infiltration by innumerable, small,pale deposits of lymphomatous tissue. This is the typical appearance of disseminated lymphoma, the liver being involved in up to 50% of cases of either the Hodgkin's or non-Hodgkin's type. Very rarely a lymphoma may arise primarily in the liver.

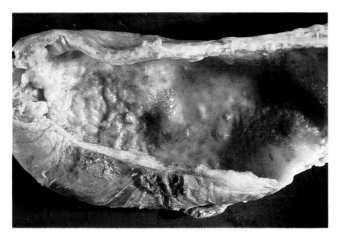

Fig.4.23 Acute cholecystitis. This gallbladder has been opened to show intense congestion and ulceration of the surface epithelium. The serosal surface is also congested and the remnants of a fibrino-purulent exudate are visible. Acute cholecystitis is seen most often in association with gallstones (see Fig.4.25), particularly if the cystic duct is obstructed. Occasional cases may occur in typhoid fever or septicaemia. Possible complications include perforation and peritonitis.

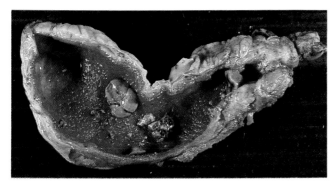

Fig.4.24 Chronic cholecystitis. The gallbladder is very shrunken and its wall is thickened and fibrotic. The mucosal surface is congested and there are several small intraluminal gallstones. These appearances represent the effects of prolonged, usually intermittent, attacks of acute cholecystitis. As such, the coexistence of gallstones is extremely common.

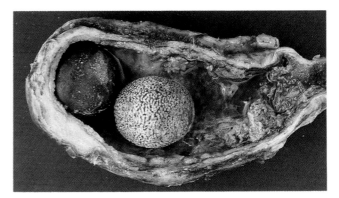

Fig.4.25 Cholelithiasis. This opened gallbladder contains two large mixed gallstones. Note the marked thickening of the gallbladder wall and the stigmata of acute inflammation of the mucosa. Gallstones are extremely common and may be of cholesterol, bile pigment or mixed type. Adults, particularly women, are most often affected. Alterations in the bile content are probably the most important aetiological factors. Complications include cholecystitis, biliary obstruction, cholangitis, and stricture of the common bile duct.

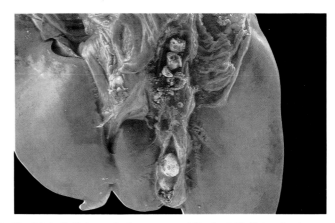

Fig.4.26 Gallstones in the common bile duct. Multiple mixed gallstones are visible within both the gallbladder (below) and the grossly dilated cystic and common bile ducts. The passage of such stones into the bile ducts may result in biliary colic or obstructive jaundice, sometimes complicated by ascending infection. Damage to the duct wall can lead to stricture formation or, occasionally, ulceration into the duodenum which may later be succeeded by gallstone ileus.

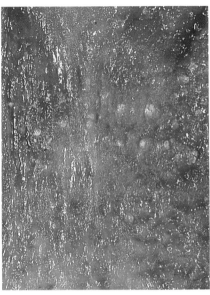

Fig.4.27 Cholesterolosis. The mucosa of the gallbladder is rather congested and is studded with multiple small, yellow flecks; this appearance is known as the 'strawberry' gallbladder. Cholesterolosis is a very common condition characterised by deposition of lipid beneath the mucosa. It rarely causes symptoms and is thought to be due to a localised abnormality of cholesterol metabolism or absorption.

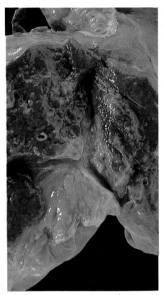

Fig.4.29 Cholangiocarcinoma. Arising at the confluence of the right and left main hepatic ducts is a pale, locally infiltrative tumour. Each of the ducts is markedly dilated. Cholangio-carcinoma (primary bile duct carcinoma) is more commonly extrahepatic than intrahepatic in origin. This tumour typically arises in late adult life, in either sex, and shows no association with cholelithiasis (cf. carcinoma of the gallbladder). In some Orientals, biliary infestation with the fluke *Clonorchis sinensis* is a predisposing factor.

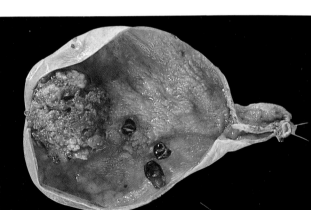

Fig.4.28 Carcinoma of gallbladder. This dilated gallbladder has been opened to show a fungating, partly papillary tumour arising in the fundus. In the body are three small pigment stones. Adeno-carcinoma of the gallbladder is uncommon and occurs most often in old age, predominantly in females. In the majority of cases there is a long-standing history of preceding cholelithiasis and cholecystitis. Invasion of the adjacent liver is an early feature, often resulting in inoperability and a poor prognosis.

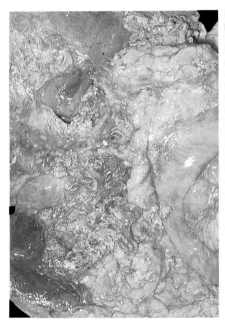

Fig.4.30 Acute pancreatitis. Between the porta hepatis (above) and an adjacent loop of small bowel there is extensive necrosis of mesenteric fat, the greyish areas re-presenting necrotic pancreatic tissue. Acute pancreatitis is relatively common and is most often associated with alcohol abuse or biliary tract disease, such as choleli-thiasis. Middle-aged adults are typically affected and the pathological features are attributable to extensive destruction by released pancreatic enzymes.

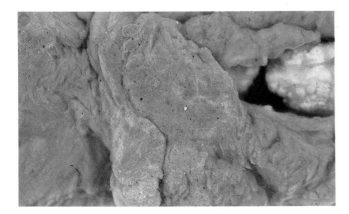

Fig.4.31 Chronic pancreatitis. The pancreatic tissue shows marked irregular scarring; the pancreatic duct (right) is dilated and contains a pale calculus. Chronic pancreatitis may take two forms: the relapsing type due to repeated acute attacks and the de novo chronic type. Both are significantly related to alcohol abuse although there may be coexistent duct obstruction or dysfunction. It is unclear whether stone formation predisposes to, or is a consequence of, chronic pancreatitis.

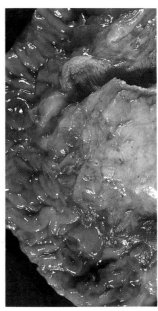

Fig.4.33 Carcinoma of the head of the pancreas. In the concavity of this loop of duodenum, the head of the pancreas is enlarged and totally replaced by a pale mass of tumour, just above which the grossly dilated (opened) common bile duct is evident. Up to 70% of exocrine pancreatic adenocarcinomas arise in the head of the gland; males are most often affected, usually in the 6th and 7th decades. Hepatobiliary failure with jaundice, due to bile duct obstruction, inoperability and the complications of radical surgery result in a very poor prognosis, although metastases may be absent or minimal.

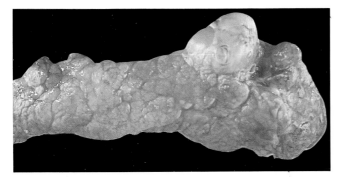

Fig.4.32 Congenital pancreatic cyst. Projecting from the superior surface of this otherwise normal pancreas is a small, smooth multiloculated cyst. Pancreatic cysts may be congenital (often associated with renal polycystic disease or cerebral angiomas), acquired due to pancreatic duct obstruction (retention cyst), neoplastic (being either a cystadenoma or cystadenocarcinoma) or false in nature (walled-off necrotic areas complicating acute pancreatitis - pseudocyst).

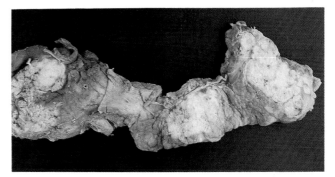

Fig.4.34 Malignant islet cell tumour. This pancreas contains multiple, irregular pale masses of tumour, the largest of which is in the tail of the gland. The majority of islet cell tumours are, in fact, benign, the commonest being an adenoma of β cells giving rise to hyperinsulinism. Other adenomas may secrete glucagon (α cells), somatostatin (δ cells), gastrin (perhaps from δ cells), pancreatic polypeptide or vasoactive intestinal polypeptide. Islet cell tumours may form part of the Type I Multiple Endocrine Neoplasia Syndrome. Up to 60% of gastrin-secreting tumours are malignant. In this case there has been extensive intrapancreatic spread.

5 Breast

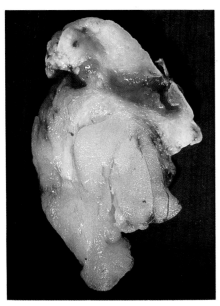

**Fig.5.1
Mammillary fistula.**
This section through areolar skin and adjacent breast tissue shows an inflamed fistulous tract, communicating with a small abscess cavity (left). Such a fistula most often occurs as a complication of recurrent pyogenic mastitis and may be associated with duct obstruction or duct ectasia. Lactation is a common predisposing factor.

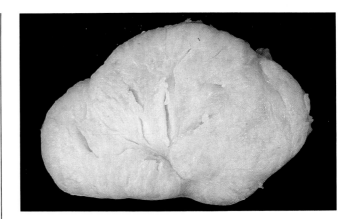

Fig.5.3 Fibroadenoma. The specimen consists of a well-circumscribed, pale, lobulated tumour which has been 'shelled out' from the adjacent breast tissue at operation. Fibroadenomas are extremely common benign neoplasms, which may be multiple and typically arise between the menarche and the age of 30. They are mobile and rubbery, whence the term 'breast mouse', and are not related to the development of breast cancer.

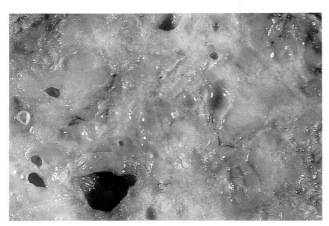

Fig.5.2 Fibrocystic disease. This breast tissue has been sectioned to show diffuse fibrosis and multiple cysts of variable size. This condition is extremely common, is often bilateral and usually affects females in the 4th and 5th decades. It is probably due to a disordered or imbalanced response to endogenous sex hormones. Only in those cases showing marked epithelial hyperplasia (epitheliosis) is there thought to be an increased risk of breast carcinoma.

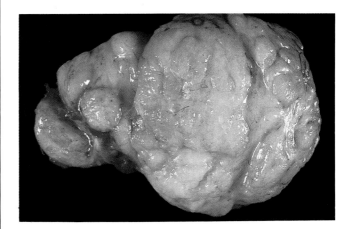

Fig.5.4 Fibroadenoma. This is a rather larger example than Fig.5.3 and demonstrates particularly well the characteristic lobulation that these tumours often show. The lobules are clearly demarcated by pale bands of fibrous tissue. It is worth noting that the historical division of fibroadenomas into intracanalicular and pericanalicular subtypes is probably spurious, since on histological grounds the two patterns almost invariably coexist.

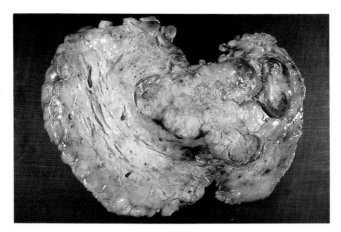

Fig.5.5 Giant fibroadenoma (Phyllodes tumour). Within the breast tissue is a large, lobulated mass showing myxoid, haemorrhagic and cystic foci. These tumours are relatively uncommon, occur predominantly in the 5th and 6th decades and may attain a great size. They are probably unrelated to the more common fibroadenomas (see page 45). Despite their obsolete name, cystosarcoma phyllodes, only about 5% behave in a malignant fashion.

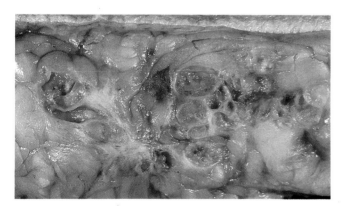

Fig.5.6 Duct papillomata. A transverse section through this breast tissue shows a collection of cystically dilated ducts, in many of which the lumen is obstructed by soft, brownish, papillary tissue. These represent multiple duct papillomata which typically arise in a major lactiferous duct, near the nipple. Duct papillomata are, however, usually solitary, arise in middle-aged women and are uncommon benign lesions. They frequently give rise to a blood-stained discharge, causing clinical confusion with carcinoma.

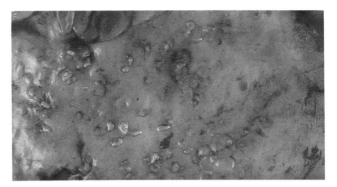

Fig.5.7 Intraduct carcinoma. On the cut surface of this breast tissue multiple small ducts, obstructed by pale tumour, are visible. The tumour appears to ooze out, rather like toothpaste - an appearance also known as comedo carcinoma. Intraduct carcinoma represents the pre-invasive stage of breast cancer of duct origin: there is also an intralobular equivalent which may be bilateral in up to 40% of patients. Excision at this stage, in the absence of histological invasion, is curative.

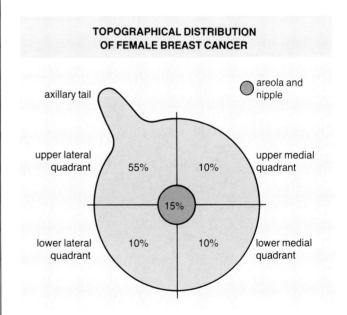

Fig.5.8 Topographical distribution of female breast carcinoma.

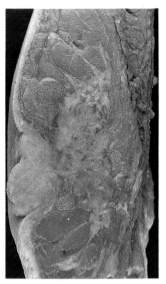

Fig.5.9 Scirrhous adenocarcinoma. A cross-section through the breast shows an irregular, pale, stippled mass beneath the retracted nipple. Note the claw-like extensions of tumour and fibrous tissue in the adjacent fat. This is the commonest macroscopical variant of breast cancer, which occurs in about 6% of females, usually in the 5th/6th decades, and is by far the commonest malignancy in women. The aetiology is uncertain but lack of previous lactation, geographical factors and epitheliosis seem to be important: 90% are of duct origin and 10% lobular. Lymph node involvement is the most important prognostic factor. 5-year-survival is only 30%, largely due to failure in early diagnosis.

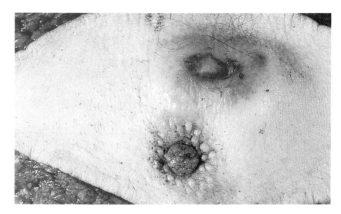

Fig.5.11 Ulcerated adenocarcinoma. Above the nipple, the skin of this mastectomy specimen is raised and ulcerated by an underlying carcinoma. Local invasion of the skin by breast cancer is common and may confer a worse prognosis. Cutaneous involvement, locally or at a distant site, may also occur due to lymphatic or haematogenous spread.

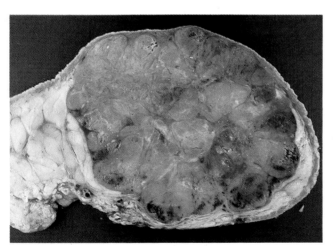

Fig.5.10 Encephaloid adenocarcinoma. Much of this breast is replaced by a large, fairly well circumscribed, lobulated tumour showing focal cystic and haemorrhagic change. The cut surface resembles cerebral tissue. This macroscopical variant of breast cancer accounts for about 8% of cases and most often represents the medullary or colloid histological subtypes. Both these types carry a better than average prognosis.

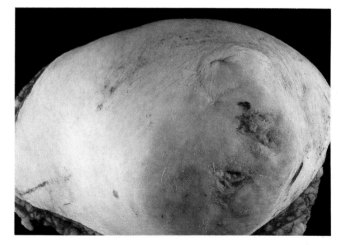

Fig.5.12 Carcinoma with nipple retraction. The breast is severely distorted by a large underlying carcinoma, with resulting ulceration and local inflammation. Above the tumour, the nipple is totally retracted within the areola (arrowed). Recent onset of nipple retraction may be a very useful clinical sign in the diagnosis of breast cancer, particularly if the underlying tumour is small or impalpable.

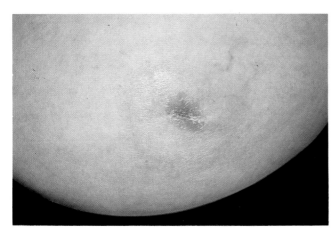

Fig.5.13 Paget's disease of the nipple. The nipple is eroded and shows an eczematous rash which extends to involve the areola. Mammary Paget's disease represents infiltration of the skin by an underlying ductal adenocarcinoma, which is present in every case (even if impalpable). This is a feature of only about 1% of breast cancers. Skin biopsy is mandatory in all adult cases of eczema of the nipple since mistaken treatment for dermatitis will delay definitive surgery and may impair the prognosis.

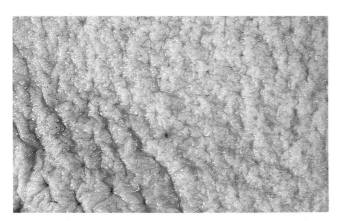

Fig.5.14 Peau d'orange. The skin of this breast is irregularly dimpled and pitted, bearing a superficial resemblance to orange peel. This appearance is seen in advanced breast cancer and is due to local lymphoedema, resulting from lymphatic obstruction by invasive tumour cells. Pitting occurs because mammary skin is tethered by innumerable sweat glands.

LYMPHATIC SPREAD OF BREAST CANCER

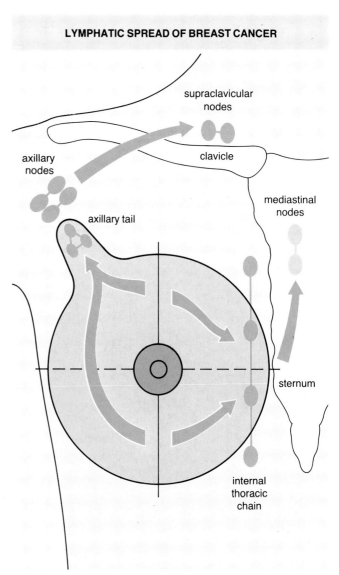

Fig.5.15 Lymphatic spread of breast cancer. Lymph node metastases are present at the time of diagnosis in up to 60% of cases. Local retrograde spread within superficial lymphatics may give rise to peau d'orange (see Fig.5.14) or carcinoma-en-cuirasse.

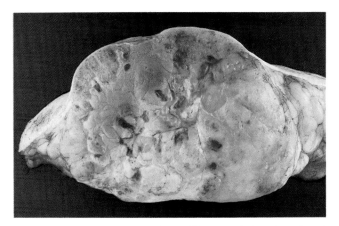

Fig.5.16 Non-Hodgkin's lymphoma. The breast is largely replaced by a pale, focally haemorrhagic mass which is well circumscribed and not dissimilar to an encephaloid carcinoma in appearance. Primary Hodgkin's or non-Hodgkin's lymphoma of the breast is uncommon but well recognised and is often succeeded by systemic dissemination. The breast may also be secondarily involved by a primary neoplasm arising in lymphoid tissue.

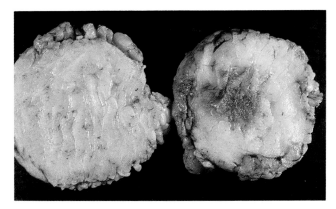

Fig.5.17 Gynaecomastia. These are bilateral subcutaneous mastectomy specimens from a young man: each shows very marked hypertrophy of fibrofatty breast tissue. Gynaecomastia (enlargement of the male breast) may be physiological, as sometimes occurs at puberty or in old age, or pathological. Causes of the latter include endocrine disturbances, a variety of drugs,(e.g. cimetidine), Klinefelter's syndrome and testicular or adrenal tumours. This condition is unrelated to the development of male breast cancer.

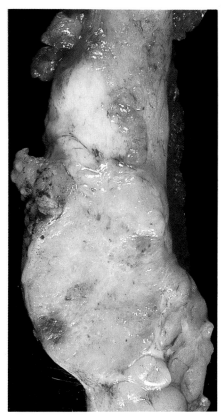

Fig.5.18 Male breast carcinoma. A section through this male breast shows diffuse replacement by pale tumour with tethering of the overlying nipple, (centre left). The pectoral muscle (right) is not involved. Male breast cancer is about 100 times less common than its female counterpart and tends to affect rather older patients. Histologically, the same types are seen in both groups but the prognosis in men is even worse, probably because extensive local invasion occurs at an earlier stage due to the small size of the male breast.

6 Lymphoreticular System

CAUSES OF SPLENOMEGALY

VASCULAR CONGESTION	Congestive cardiac failure	
	Portal hypertension	
INFECTIVE	Pyogenic	bacterial septicaemia
	Non-pyogenic	TB, viral, fungal, parasitic (malaria)
HAEMATOLOGICAL	Abnormal RBC's (haemolytic anaemias)	
	Extramedullary haemopoiesis	
METABOLIC	Lipid storage diseases	
	Glycogen storage diseases	
NEOPLASTIC	Primary	haemangioma
	Secondary	lymphoma
		leukaemia
		carcinoma
MISCELLANEOUS	Amyloidosis	
	Sarcoidosis	

SPLENOMEGALY CLASSIFIED BY WEIGHT

MILD <500g	Acute infection or congestion
MODERATE 500-1000g	Chronic infection or congestion
	Haematological causes
	Amyloidosis
MASSIVE >1000g	Lymphoma, leukaemia or myeloproliferative disorder
	Storage diseases

Fig.6.1 Causes of splenomegaly.

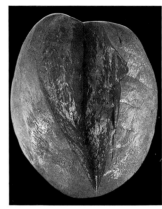

Fig.6.2 **Passive venous congestion.** This enlarged spleen, weighing 740g, is very firm (retaining its shape despite being sliced) and is rather rounded in appearance (being known as a 'cricket ball spleen'). Passive venous congestion is the commonest cause of splenomegaly: there is usually only mild enlargement (most often as a consequence of congestive cardiac failure) but greater expansion (as here) may be seen in chronic portal hypertension (e.g. due to hepatic cirrhosis).

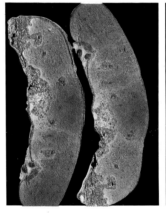

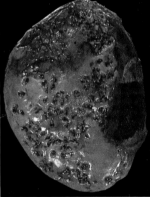

Fig.6.3 **Splenic infarction.** Almost the entire spleen shows dull reddish infarction, only those areas with a granular cut surface being spared. Thrombus is clearly visible occluding the splenic artery. Splenic infarction may be embolic in origin, or due to local thrombosis (e.g. complicating atheroma, sickle cell anaemia or polyarteritis) or due to torsion. Small infarcts are also commonly seen in almost any case of moderate or massive splenomegaly.

Fig.6.4 **Chronic perisplenitis.** The splenic capsule is covered in dense, irregular, hyalinised, fibrous tissue. This appearance, known as 'sugar-icing' spleen, may be seen in any case of long-standing splenomegaly or associated with chronic pleural inflammation. Acute perisplenitis, characterised by a serosal fibrinous exudate, may occur in cases of septicaemia or overlying a splenic infarct.

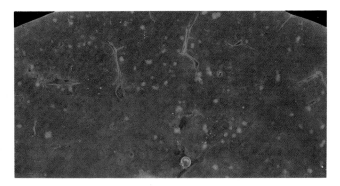

Fig.6.5 Miliary tuberculosis. Scattered throughout the splenic parenchyma are multiple, tiny, pale nodules resembling millet seed (hence the name). Miliary tuberculosis represents haematogenous spread of infection, most often from a primary focus in the lung (see Chapter 2). This vascular dissemination results from encroachment and ulceration of the infective process through a vessel wall: this leads to intrapulmonary spread, in addition to involvement of other organs such as the liver, bone marrow and kidneys.

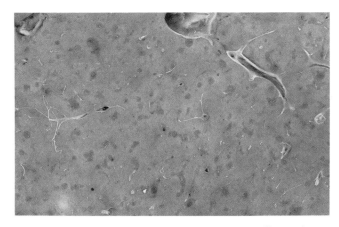

Fig.6.7 Amyloidosis. The splenic cut surface has a diffuse pale, waxy appearance. The spleen is more often involved in secondary, rather than primary, amyloidosis as may be seen in any long-standing infective or inflammatory condition. Moderate splenomegaly commonly results.

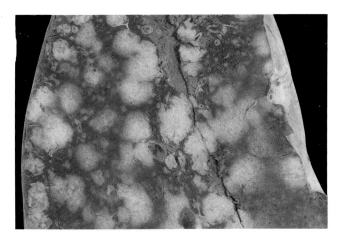

Fig.6.6 Sarcoidosis. Scattered throughout the splenic parenchyma are coarse pale nodules, arising mainly in the white pulp. Sarcoidosis is an idiopathic, granulomatous, chronic inflammatory disorder, which is commonest in young adults. Lymphoid tissue throughout the body is predominantly affected, although palpable splenomegaly is seen in only about 20% of cases. Typically, the lungs are also involved and patients often present with respiratory symptoms; pulmonary interstitial fibrosis is an occasional complication.

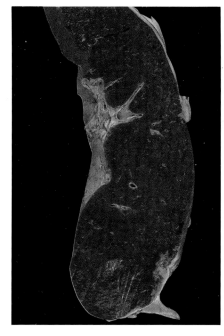

Fig.6.8 Myelofibrosis. This spleen is massively enlarged, weighing 3,175g, and is uniformly deep red in colour. The myeloproliferative disorders and chronic leukaemias are the commonest causes of massive splenomegaly. In the myeloproliferative cases this enlargement is due to the development of extramedullary haemopoiesis (an integral part of the disease process, not secondary to marrow destruction), while in the leukaemias, there is extensive infiltration by neoplastic cells.

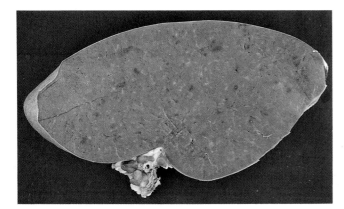

Fig.6.9 Chronic lymphatic leukaemia. This spleen is uniformly enlarged and rather paler than normal. Smooth lymphadenopathy is also visible at the hilum. Chronic lymphatic leukaemia is not uncommon and affects mainly the elderly with a predominance in men. There is usually a massive circulating lymphocytosis and generalised lymphadenopathy. Splenomegaly, as in chronic myeloid leukaemia, may be massive and the long-term prognosis is generally poor, although in the elderly life expectancy may not be affected.

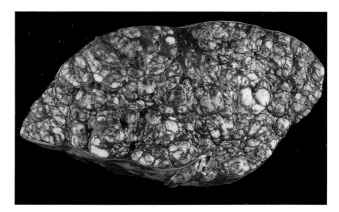

Fig.6.11 Non-Hodgkin's lymphoma. This greatly enlarged spleen is diffusely replaced by coarse nodular deposits of pale tumour. Splenic involvement is very common in any non-Hodgkin's lymphoma but particularly in the follicular (Lukes and Collins) subtypes. Two points are worth remembering in any patient with lymphoma: (1) the resultant splenomegaly may cause destruction of red cells, white cells or platelets (hypersplenism) of itself, and (2) splenomegaly may be due to recurrent or chronic coexistent infection.

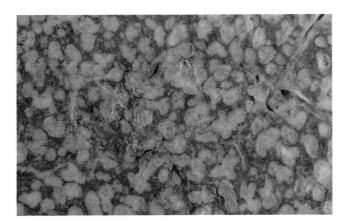

Fig.6.10 Hodgkin's disease. The white pulp is expanded and replaced by innumerable, irregular, pale deposits of tumour. This is the classical appearance of so-called 'salami' spleen in Hodgkin's disease, although almost any macroscopical distribution (as in non-Hodgkin's lymphoma) may be seen. Splenic involvement occurs in up to 50% of cases of Hodgkin's disease and is most often detected at staging laparotomy.

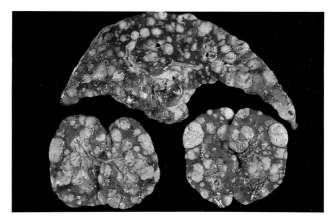

Fig.6.12 Burkitt's lymphoma. Both kidneys and the liver are extensively replaced by multiple large lymphomatous deposits. Burkitt's lymphoma, a specific subtype of non-Hodgkin's lymphoma, is typically a disease of children, most often seen in equatorial Africa. It is caused by Epstein-Barr virus and endemic malaria acts as a co-factor. It has a peculiar tendency to arise in the jaw, ovary, adrenal or kidney.

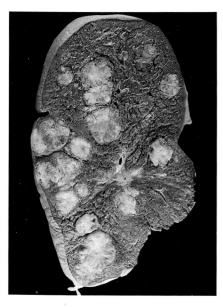

Fig.6.13 Secondary carcinoma. Within the spleen are multiple, pale, umbilicated metastases. Splenic metastases, surprisingly, are relatively uncommon, being macroscopically evident in only about 5% of cases of disseminated cancer examined at post mortem. The most frequently responsible primary sites are the lung, breast, cutaneous malignant melanoma and ovary.

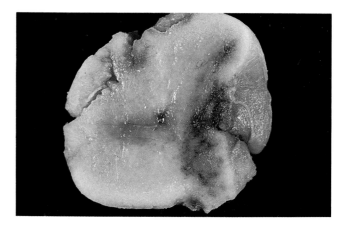

Fig.6.15 Sarcoidosis. This mediastinal lymph node shows smooth, yellowish enlargement. Small amounts of anthracotic pigment are visible on the right. While sarcoidosis is the commonest cause of bilateral pulmonary hilar lymphadenopathy, lymph nodes at any site may be affected. Other organs that are commonly involved include skin (lupus pernio), liver, muscle, eyes or bone.

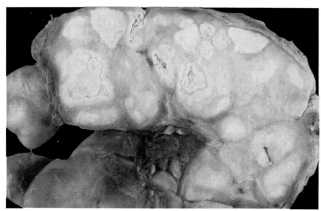

Fig.6.14 Tuberculous lymphadenopathy. These lymph nodes are densely adherent to one another and their cut surfaces show diffuse, irregular, caseous necrosis. Tuberculous infection in lymph nodes is usually seen in the regional nodes which drain the primary site of infection, for example in the mediastinum, mesentery or neck. Atypical Mycobacteria may produce a similar picture. Healing often leads to dystrophic calcification, which may be an incidental radiological finding.

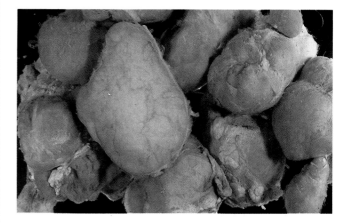

Fig.6.16 Hodgkin's disease. This group of lymph nodes each show rubbery, smooth enlargement but have remained discrete (cf. tuberculosis). The cut surface is uniform and yellowish-white. Hodgkin's disease, a lymphoma of uncertain histogenesis, shows a predilection for males and has a peak incidence in the 2nd/3rd and 6th/7th decades. The Rye histological classification and Ann Arbor staging system correlate well with prognosis. There is epidemiological evidence (case-clustering) of an infective aetiology.

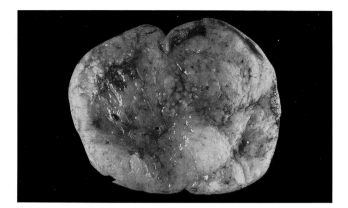

Fig.6.17 Non-Hodgkin's lymphoma. This lymph node is smoothly enlarged and has a nodular, and in places almost follicular, cut surface. Non-Hodgkin's lymphoma is more common than Hodgkin's disease and is particularly prevalent in the elderly. There may be preceding autoimmune disease or iatrogenic immunosuppression in some cases. There are several complex systems of histological classification, which are a source of confusion to many; those of Kiel or Rappaport are probably the most used.

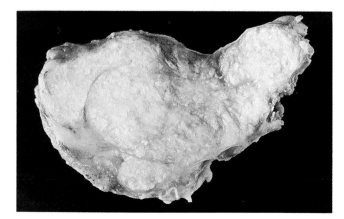

Fig.6.18 Secondary carcinoma. These lymph nodes, which are closely apposed to one another, are diffusely replaced and expanded by pale, rather granular tumour. Metastatic tumour is by far the commonest source of neoplastic lymphadenopathy, most particularly from carcinomas rather than sarcomas, which tend more to haematogenous spread. Lymph node metastases usually imply a worse prognosis than if the tumour is confined to its primary site.

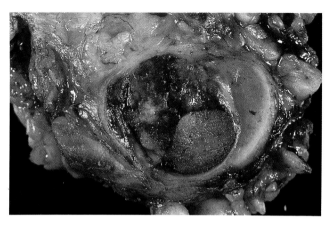

Fig.6.19 Metastatic malignant melanoma. This lymph node contains a large, well circumscribed deposit of deeply-pigmented, focally necrotic tumour. A rim of uninvolved nodal tissue is visible on the right. Malignant melanoma is particularly prone to lymphatic invasion and lymph node involvement is a common finding at presentation.

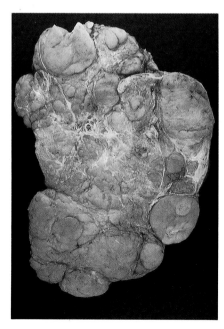

Fig.6.20 Thymoma. The thymus is greatly enlarged and is replaced by an encapsulated, multilobulated pinkish mass. The tumour lobules are separated by bands of fibrous tissue. Thymomas are uncommon, arise most often in middle age and are slow-growing, radio-sensitive tumours with a generally good prognosis. Up to a third of cases may be associated with another systemic illness, in particular myaesthenia gravis or systemic lupus erythematosus.

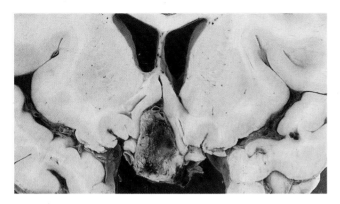

Fig.7.1 Pituitary adenoma. Arising in the pituitary fossa is a well circumscribed, rather haemorrhagic tumour. Small, non-functioning pituitary adenomas are not uncommon. Symptomatic neoplasms, which are less frequent, are most often composed of chromophobe cells (60%) or acidophils (30%): basophil adenomas are very rare. Such tumours may arise at any age and produce either local pressure effects (e.g. bitemporal hemianopia) or endocrine effects, most commonly due to the excessive secretion of prolactin or growth hormone. Pituitary adenomas may also be seen in Type I Multiple Endocrine Neoplasia Syndrome (Werner).

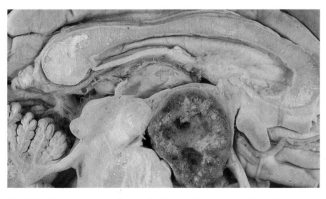

Fig.7.2 Craniopharyngioma. Arising in the region of the pituitary is a large, well circumscribed, tumour, with a variegated cut surface, which is compressing the optic chiasma anteriorly and the third ventricle superiorly. Craniopharyngiomas are traditionally held to arise from Rathke's pouch and are usually suprasellar in location. They are slow-growing lesions which present most often in childhood, usually due to pressure on the pituitary or optic tracts. They very commonly undergo cystic change or calcification.

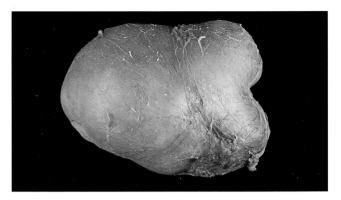

Fig.7.3 Thyroglossal cyst. This smooth, multilocular cyst contains clear, yellowish fluid and measures about 4 cm in maximum diameter. Such cysts represent vestigial remnants of the thyroglossal duct, along which the thyroid migrates *in utero* from the base of the tongue to its normal position. They may present at any age and are usually found in the midline of the neck, adjacent to the hyoid bone.

CLASSIFICATION OF THYROID ENLARGEMENT	
HYPERTHYROID	Graves' disease
	Multinodular goitre with toxic nodule
	Early Hashimoto's disease
EUTHYROID	Multinodular goitre
	Endemic colloid goitre
	Adenoma
	Dyshormonogenesis
	Carcinoma primary secondary
	Lymphoma
	De Quervain's thyroiditis
HYPOTHYROID	End-stage multinodular goitre
	Chronic Hashimoto's disease
	Endemic cretinism

Fig.7.4 Classification of thyroid enlargement.

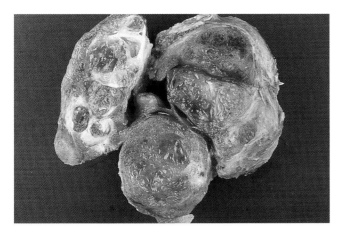

Fig.7.5   Multinodular goitre. The thyroid is distorted by multiple nodules of varying size, some of which contain colloid while others have undergone calcification and cystic change. Fibrosis is also apparent, particularly in the left upper pole. Multinodular goitres, which are quite common, represent the end stage of a diffuse non-toxic goitre: the latter may be endemic, due to iodine deficiency, or sporadic, due to environmental or genetic factors. Patients with multinodular goitre are usually euthyroid but may sometimes develop autonomous toxic nodules.

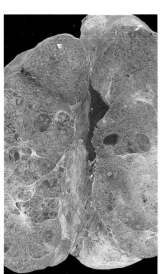

Fig.7.6   Colloid goitre. The thyroid is massively enlarged by multiple diffuse nodules, some of which are 'meaty' in appearance while others appear cystic or colloid-filled. While this appearance may represent the early stages of a diffuse non-toxic goitre due to any cause (i.e. prior to the development of in-volutional or degenerative changes), diffuse colloid goitres are most often endemic due to iodine deficiency (particularly in the drinking water). This is commonest in mountainous areas (e.g. the Alps or Himalayas) and was at one time a problem along the Pennines in this country ('Derbyshire neck').

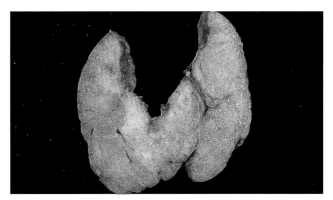

Fig.7.7   Graves' disease. The thyroid is diffusely and smoothly enlarged; the cut surface has a 'beefy' appearance. Graves' disease (diffuse toxic goitre) is commonest in young women and is an auto-immune disease, the most important autoantibodies found being those that mimic the action of TSH. Affected individuals are thyrotoxic and may show associated ophthalmopathy, pretibial myxoedema and enlargement of lymphoid tissues. This condition is closely related to Hashimoto's disease and, if treated surgically, some patients may develop hypothyroidism.

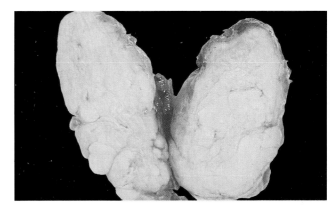

Fig.7.8   Hashimoto's disease. This thyroid is also diffusely and smoothly enlarged but the cut surface has a pale appearance (likened to normal pancreas). Hashimoto's disease is another auto-immune disease which shows a very marked predilection for young adult females, and results in autoantibody-mediated destruction of follicular cells. Patients may also have coexistent pernicious anaemia, Sjögren's syndrome or Addison's disease. At least 50% eventually become hypothyroid.

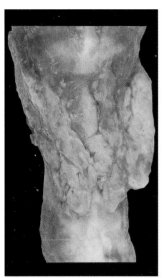

Fig.7.9 Primary myxoedema.
This thyroid, shown in situ with the trachea, is markedly shrunken, pale and fibrotic. Primary hypothyroidism in adults is usually due to chronic auto-immune thyroiditis and probably represents end-stage Hashimoto's disease. As such, middle-aged females, some-times with other autoimmune conditions, are predominantly affected. Other causes of clinical hypothyroidism include an end-stage goitre, previous thyroidec-tomy or irradiation and, rarely, dyshormonogenesis.

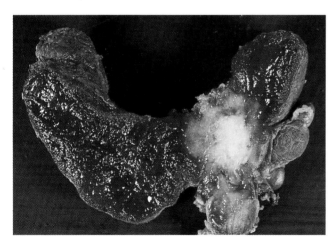

Fig.7.10 Papillary carcinoma. Arising in the right lobe of an other-wise normal thyroid is a pale, irregular neoplasm; a lymph node infiltrated by metastatic tumour is adherent to the lower pole. Papillary carcinoma accounts for about 60% of malignant thyroid neoplasms. It arises most often in young adults and shows a predilection for females. It is sometimes multicentric in origin and occasionally presents with an adjacent lymph node metastasis (known previously as the 'lateral aberrant thyroid'). The overall 5-year-survival is about 90%.

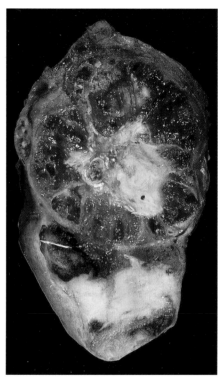

Fig.7.11 Follicular carcinoma. Within this lobe of the thyroid, distorted by a multinodular goitre, a pale infil-trative neoplasm is visible in the lower pole. Follicular car-cinoma (25% of thyroid malig-nancies) is rather commoner in females and tends to occur in middle age. Occasionally, it can be distinguished from a follicular adenoma only by microscopic evidence of vascular invasion. This tumour tends to local infiltration and vascular spread (in contrast to the lymphatic spread of papillary carcinoma) with a 5-year-survival of about 60%.

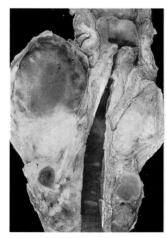

Fig.7.12 Anaplastic car-cinoma. This large, pale and focally haemorrhagic tumour has replaced most of the thyroid and is involving adjacent lymph nodes and the tracheal wall by direct extension. There is an associated florid tracheitis. Ana-plastic thyroid carcinoma, which is relatively uncommon, is virt-ually confined to the elderly. It is a rapidly progressive and lethal tumour, which tends to very extensive local invasion (often with tracheal stenosis) and is usually fatal within a year of diagnosis.

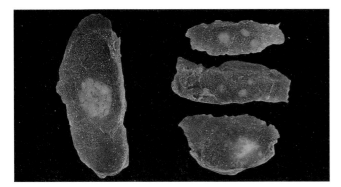

Fig.7.13 Medullary carcinoma. The cut surface of the left lobe and serial sections through the right lobe of this thyroid show multiple, reasonably circumscribed tumours of varying size. Medullary carcinoma, which is derived from parafollicular calcitonin-secreting cells, accounts for about 10% of thyroid cancers. It may be sporadic (usually in middle age) or familial (affecting younger individuals and often multifocal), forming part of the Type II Multiple Endocrine Neoplasia Syndrome (Sipple). 5-year-survival is about 50%.

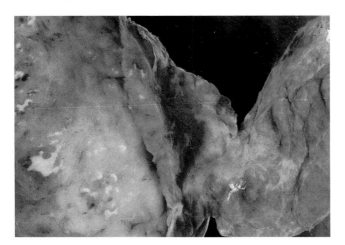

Fig.7.14 Lymphoma. Arising within and enlarging the left lobe of the thyroid is a diffuse pale neoplasm showing multifocal necrosis. Primary lymphoma of the thyroid is uncommon and is typically seen in elderly females, often with evidence of pre-existent Hashimoto's disease. Such tumours are usually non-Hodgkin's in type, although any systemically disseminated lymphoma may involve the thyroid secondarily. In general the prognosis is poor.

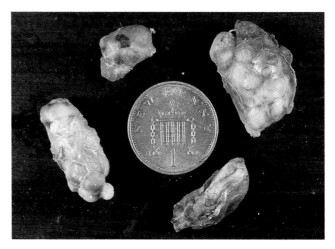

Fig.7.15 Parathyroid hyperplasia. Each of these four parathyroid glands is markedly, although rather unequally, enlarged; all have a nodular appearance. Parathyroid hyperplasia is relatively uncommon, being responsible for only about 10% of cases of hyperparathyroidism. It may be a primary idiopathic lesion, sometimes forming part of a Multiple Endocrine Neoplasia Syndrome, or it may be secondary to chronic renal failure. In long-standing cases of the latter type, autonomous true adenomas sometimes develop.

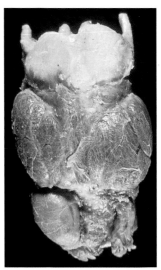

Fig.7.16 Parathyroid adenoma. Beneath the lower pole of the right lobe of the thyroid, viewed anteriorly, is a solitary, large, brownish parathyroid tumour. Parathyroid adenomas are responsible for at least 75% of cases of hyperparathyroidism and are commonest in middle age, affecting predominantly females. They are usually solitary and sometimes arise in long-standing secondary hyperparathyroidism. Elevated levels of parathormone, which more rarely are due to parathyroid carcinoma or ectopic secretion by a heterotopic malignancy, lead to nephrocalcinosis and osteitis fibrosa cystica (see Chapter 12).

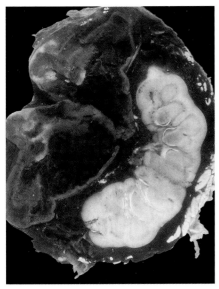

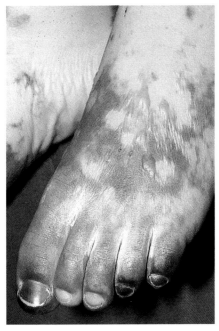

Fig.7.17 Waterhouse-Friderichsen syndrome. The adrenal gland (top), the outline of which is just visible, has been totally destroyed by extensive haemorrhage. Below, the feet of a young boy show the typical petechial rash, with cyanosis and gangrene. Waterhouse-Friderichsen syndrome refers *solely* to the occurrence of adrenal haemorrhage associated with a severe septicaemic illness. It is classically seen in children or young adults, most often with meningococcal septicaemia. The adrenal haemorrhage, which is usually fatal, is thought to result from a combination of endotoxin-induced cell damage, 'stress' and a degree of disseminated intravascular coagulation.

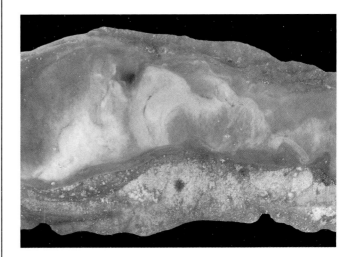

Fig.7.18 Primary Addison's disease. This adrenal gland, seen in cross-section, is markedly shrunken and thinned, measuring less than 2 cm in length. Addison's disease, or chronic adrenocortical insufficiency, is most often due to idiopathic autoimmune destruction, analagous to primary myxoedema. More than 90% of adrenocortical tissue has to be lost before the typical symptoms or electrolyte disturbances result.

Fig.7.19 Addison's disease due to tuberculosis. The cortex and medulla of this adrenal show extensive caseous necrosis and the surrounding capsule has undergone dystrophic calcification. Prior to the recognition of autoimmune disease, TB was regarded as the commonest identifiable cause of Addison's disease, although this occurrence is now rare in the Western World. However, it is typically a complication of pre-existent pulmonary infection. Other causes of Addison's disease include amyloidosis, metastatic carcinoma, haemochromatosis and histoplasmosis.

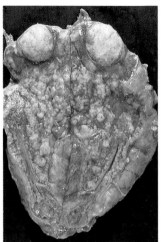

Fig.7.20 Adrenocortical nodular hyperplasia. The cortex of this adrenal gland, which has been partially bisected, contains multiple bright-yellow nodules, the largest of which is visible at the apex. Such nodular hyperplasia is idiopathic and is probably far more common than a solitary adenoma. The true incidence is, however, uncertain since these nodules are typically non-functioning and do not give rise to any endocrine disturbance. This appearance is sometimes associated with benign hypertension, an unexplained phenomenon.

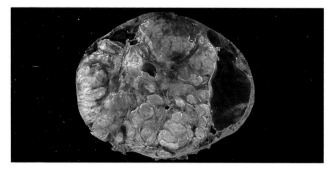

Fig.7.22 Adrenocortical carcinoma. This adrenal gland, measuring 20cm in maximum diameter, is massively enlarged by a multinodular tumour showing extensive cystic change and haemorrhage. Adrenocortical carcinoma is rare but may occur at any age. These tumours are typically non-functioning and therefore often attain a great size prior to presentation. The presence of metastases is far more reliable than the histological appearances in distinguishing malignant lesions but, in general, these latter tend to rapid and extensive haematogenous dissemination.

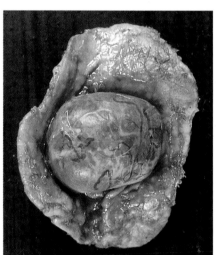 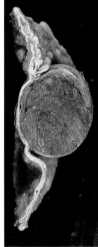

Fig.7.21 Adrenocortical adenoma. On the left, a smooth, well circumscribed tumour projects from the cortical surface of an adrenal. The same gland in cross-section (right) shows a solitary brownish lesion with marked atrophy of the adjacent cortex. Such solitary functioning adenomas, as opposed to cortical nodules (see above), are relatively uncommon but may result in Cushing's syndrome with consequent pituitary suppression (as here) or in hyperaldosteronism (Conn's syndrome).

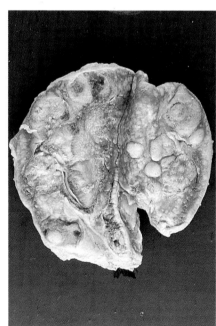

Fig.7.23 Metastatic carcinoma. This partially bisected adrenal gland is irregularly distorted by numerous nodules of pale secondary tumour, some of which show necrosis or haemorrhage. While any malignant tumour may metastasise to the adrenal, by far the commonest to do so is carcinoma of the bronchus, followed by breast carcinoma and malignant melanoma. Such spread is usually bilateral and may occasionally give rise to Addison's disease (see Figs. 7.18 & 7.19).

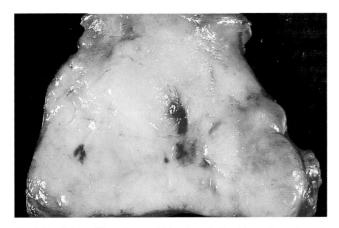

Fig.7.24 Adrenal lymphoma. This adrenal gland is totally replaced by an irregular mass of pale yellowish-pink tissue. Primary lymphoma of the adrenal gland, which is usually non-Hodgkin's in type, is extremely rare. Even secondary involvement by any histological type undergoing systemic dissemination is very uncommon.

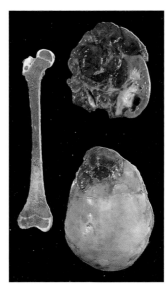

Fig.7.26 Neuroblastoma. Replacing the left adrenal (top right) is a large, multinodular haemorrhagic mass. Deposits of metastatic tumour are visible in this child's skull and femur. Neuroblastomas arise from non-chromaffin cells in the adrenal medulla (or sympathetic chain) and are seen almost solely in young children. They are highly malignant lesions, which occasionally secrete catecholamines; modern modes of treatment have led to an improved survival rate. Interestingly, lesions in the right adrenal metastasise more often to the liver, in contrast to the case here.

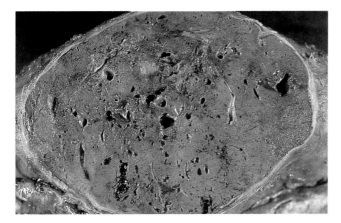

Fig.7.25 Phaeochromocytoma. The adrenal medulla is grossly expanded and replaced by a tan-coloured, rather vascular tumour showing foci of haemorrhage. The attenuated cortex is visible as a yellow rim of tissue. Phaeochromocytomas arise from chromaffin cells, typically in young adults, and may be associated with neurofibromatosis or Type II Multiple Endocrine Neoplasia Syndrome. While the vast majority are benign, they secrete excessive amounts of catecholamines, giving rise to paroxysmal hypertension. They are not uncommonly bilateral.

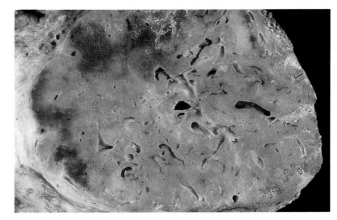

Fig.7.27 Chemodectoma. This specimen comprises a well circumscribed, brownish, vascular mass showing areas of haemorrhage. Chemodectomas are the commonest neuroendocrine tumours of the extra-adrenal paraganglionic system and may be seen at any age. They most often arise in the carotid body and are commoner in populations living at high altitude (probably as a consequence of prolonged hypoxia). Similar lesions arising in the temporal bone or at the base of the skull are known as glomus jugulare tumours. A variable number behave in a malignant fashion.

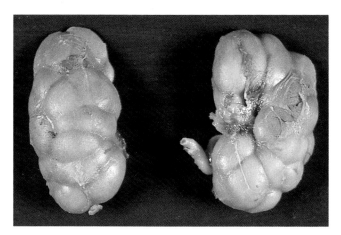

Fig.8.1 Fetal renal lobulation. These are kidneys from a stillborn infant: note the marked cortical lobulation. This appearance is entirely normal but is usually no longer apparent by one year of age. However, lobulation, if only partial, sometimes persists into adult life and it is important to recognise that such a finding is of no pathological importance.

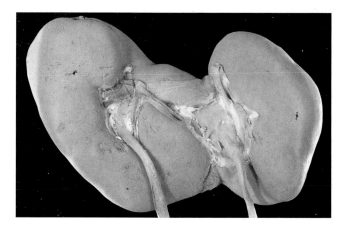

Fig.8.2 Horseshoe kidney. The kidneys are fused at their lower poles and both renal hila lie anteriorly. The isthmus of renal tissue which joins the two kidneys lay over the aorta *in vivo*. Renal fusion occurs in at least 1 in 250 individuals and results from partial failure of embryological ascent of nephrogenic tissue, followed by malrotation. Coexistent anomalies of the ureters or renal vessels are often also seen and may predispose to urinary infection or obstruction.

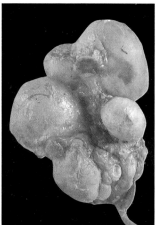

Fig.8.3 'Infantile' polycystic disease. The renal parenchyma of this adolescent's kidney is completely replaced by thin-walled cysts. Infantile polycystic disease may take a variety of forms. Classically, it has an autosomal recessive inheritance and takes a fatal course in infancy. In such cases the kidneys appear normal externally but show numerous small, radially arranged cysts on sectioning. There is always associated congenital hepatic fibrosis; in some cases (as here) the renal appearances and clinical duration may be very variable.

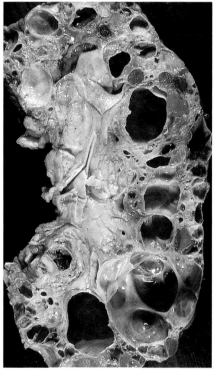

Fig.8.4 Adult polycystic disease. This kidney has been bisected through the hilum to show extensive parenchymal replacement by cysts of varying size, into some of which haemorrhage has occured. Adult polycystic disease is an autosomal dominant inherited condition; patients typically present in middle age and chronic renal failure usually supervenes thereafter. Associated hepatic or pancreatic cysts and cerebral berry aneurysms may also be found.

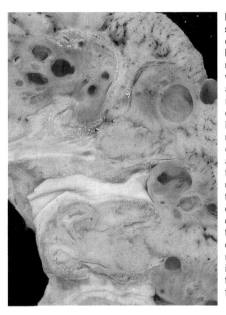

Fig.8.5 Medullary sponge kidney. The cut surface of this kidney shows multiple, smooth-walled cysts which are confined to the renal papillae. This condition, thought to be due to developmentally anomalous collecting ducts, affects males more than females and is usually detected in the 5th or 6th decades. Calculi often develop within the cysts and, in combination with recurrent urinary infection, may lead to impaired renal function.

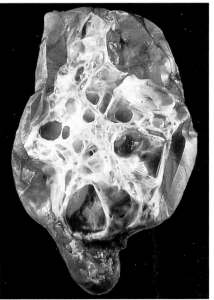

Fig.8.6 Renal dysplasia. Much, but not all, of this kidney is replaced by coarse, irregular cysts separated by broad bands of fibrous tissue. Renal dysplasia, which represents failure of nephrogenic differentiation, may affect one or both kidneys and may involve either the whole, or only part, of the kidney. Often other developmental anomalies, usually obstructive in nature, are present elsewhere in the urinary tract.

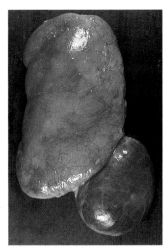

Fig.8.7 Simple renal cyst. Arising from the cortex of the lower pole of this kidney is a large, thin-walled cyst. Simple renal cysts are extremely common, particularly with advancing age, and are thought to represent the local effect of previous ischaemia or obstruction. They are usually solitary, are typically located in the cortex and are most often only about 1 cm in diameter, the example here being unusually large.

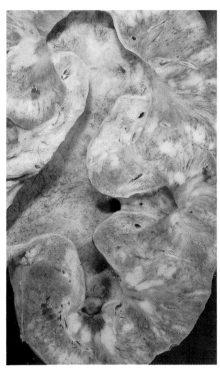

Fig.8.8 Acute pyelonephritis. This hemisected kidney shows intense congestion and innumerable, radially arranged yellow areas of suppuration and abscess formation, especially in the medulla. Acute pyelonephritis is not uncommon and is usually a consequence of ascending Gram-negative infection. Common predisposing causes include urinary obstruction, diabetes mellitus and pregnancy. In general, females are most often affected, probably as a consequence of peri-urethral contamination by faecal organisms.

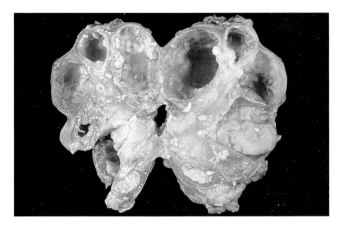

Fig.8.9 Renal tuberculosis. The parenchyma of this bisected kidney shows numerous confluent foci of caseous necrosis; there is also marked calyceal involvement with dilatation, giving rise to so-called 'pyonephrosis' (despite the absence of pus). Renal tuberculosis is often bilateral, is commonest in adult males and is usually due to haematogenous spread from primary infection elsewhere. While remaining endemic in some parts of the world, this infection is now uncommon in Caucasians.

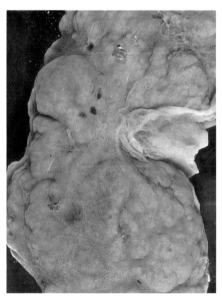

Fig.8.10 Chronic interstitial nephritis. The capsular surface of this kidney shows coarse, irregular scarring and the whole organ is rather shrunken. Chronic interstitial nephritis is the term used to describe chronic parenchymal inflammation and atrophy, which may be a consequence of various conditions including chronic suppurative pyelonephritis, long-standing ischaemia or obstruction and analgesic nephropathy.

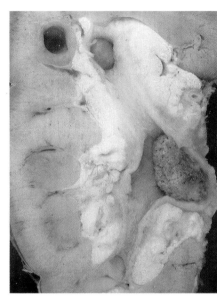

Fig.8.11 Renal calculus. Lying within the renal pelvis is an irregular, ovoid stone. Surprisingly, there is no evidence of hydronephrosis. Calculi in the urinary tract are common, are seen most frequently in the kidney and usually present in adulthood. Predisposing causes include urinary obstruction, an elevated urinary concentration of the relevant constituent or altered urinary pH facilitating crystal precipitation.

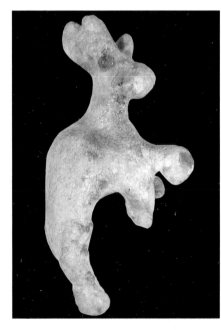

Fig.8.12 Staghorn renal calculus. This stone has a branched appearance (resembling the antlers of a stag) and formed an accurate cast of the pelvicalyceal system and upper ureter from which it was removed. Staghorn calculi are typically composed of calcium phosphate (the commonest constituent of renal stones) but may also be made up of 'triple' phosphate or cystine. Complications of urinary lithiasis include obstruction, infection and haematuria.

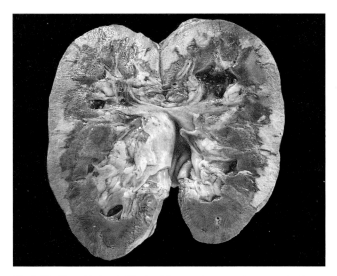

Fig.8.13 Renal infarct. Much of the renal cortex shows marked pallor, although the lower pole is spared. The margins of the infarct are hyperaemic. This is an unusually large renal infarct, small wedge-shaped lesions being more common. Infarction of the kidney is nearly always due to arterial occlusion by embolism or thrombosis. Emboli are usually cardiac in origin and, if derived from the vegetations of bacterial endocarditis, may give rise to septic infarcts with abscess formation.

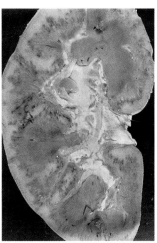

Fig.8.14 Renal cortical necrosis. The entire renal cortex is pale and necrotic, while the corticomedullary junction is congested. Renal cortical necrosis is usually a consequence of disseminated intravascular coagulation, as may occur in antepartum placental haemorrhage, septicaemic illnesses or severe trauma. Acute renal failure rapidly supervenes and the prognosis is generally poor. Multifocal cortical necrosis may also be seen in the haemolytic-uraemic syndrome.

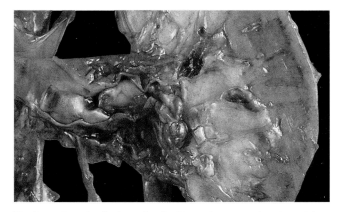

Fig.8.15 Renal vein thrombosis. The entire kidney is pale and the main renal vein is completely occluded by organised thrombus. While renal vein thrombosis may be acute in neonates (giving rise to red infarction), in older individuals the onset is usually gradual, resulting in oedema and tubular atrophy. In the latter group, thrombosis is usually secondary to chronic glomerulonephritis or amyloidosis and the outcome is most often fatal.

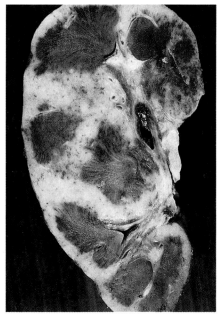

Fig.8.16 Acute transplant rejection. The renal cortex is pale, swollen and shows small petechial haemorrhages. The medulla is very intensely congested. This is a classical example of acute rejection which usually occurs within a year of transplantation and is most often due to the development of recipient anti-graft antibodies. Rejection may also be hyperacute, due to pre-existent sensitisation to donor antigens, or chronic (see Fig.8.17).

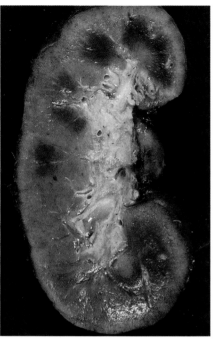

Fig.8.17 Chronic transplant rejection. This kidney shows a non-specific, congested and rather mottled appearance. Chronic rejection of a renal transplant tends to occur several months, or even years, after grafting and is often characterised by the asymptomatic development of either hypertension or the nephrotic syndrome. It is thought to be due to chronic low-grade arterial damage (due to deposition of microthrombi), combined with complex-mediated glomerulonephritis and tubular atrophy.

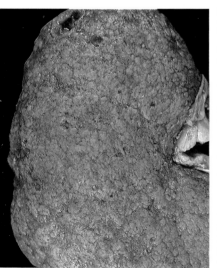

Fig.8.18 Essential hypertension. This kidney is slightly shrunken and the capsular surface shows fine granular scarring, along with several small simple cysts. Renal changes in benign hypertension are largely microscopic and are principally ischaemic in nature. There is usually little if any impairment of renal function but up to 5% of patients develop malignant hypertension with subsequent renal failure.

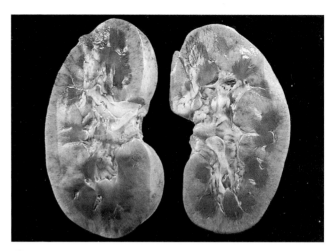

Fig.8.19 Acute proliferative glomerulonephritis. This bisected kidney is rather swollen and there are petechial haemorrhages in the cortex. Acute proliferative glomerulonephritis is fairly uncommon, occurs predominantly in children and usually follows a group A streptococcal upper respiratory infection. It is thought to be due to desposition of circulating immune complexes and often gives rise to the nephritic syndrome. In the majority of cases spontaneous recovery occurs.

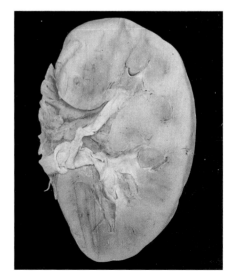

Fig.8.20 Membranous glomerulonephritis. This kidney has been sectioned to show extreme cortical pallor, oedema and blurring of the corticomedullary junction. Membranous glomerulonephritis is an idiopathic condition, due to the deposition of circulating immune complexes, which typically presents in adulthood. Up to 70% of patients develop chronic renal failure.

CAUSES OF NEPHROTIC SYNDROME

PRIMARY RENAL DISEASE	Glomerulo-nephritis	minimal change
		membranous
		membrano-proliferative
		focal segmental glomerulo-sclerosis
	Congenital	Alport's syndrome
	Renal vein thrombosis	
SECONDARY RENAL DISEASE	Diabetes mellitus	
	Amyloidosis	
	Systemic lupus erythematosus	
	Drugs	penicillamine
	Infections	hepatitis B
		malaria
	Malignancy	lymphoma
		bronchial carcinoma

Fig.8.21   Causes of nephrotic syndrome.

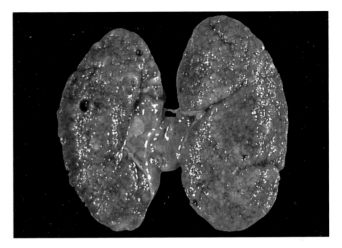

Fig.8.22   Chronic glomerulonephritis. This kidney is shrunken and shows severe granular scarring of the cortical surface. Chronic glomerulonephritis is the non-specific end-stage form of many primary glomerular diseases. However, in a proportion of cases, the primary initiating episode has passed unnoticed. Chronic renal failure always develops and, without dialysis or transplantation, death is invariable.

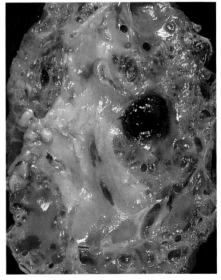

Fig.8.23   Chronic glomerulonephritis with secondary cystic change. In addition to being markedly shrunken and scarred, the renal parenchyma contains innumerable small cysts. This appearance is now well recognised in patients who have been maintained on long-term dialysis for chronic renal failure. It is thought to be a secondary phenomenon, perhaps related to renal tubular obstruction.

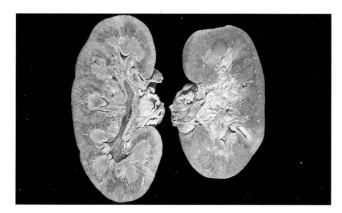

Fig.8.24 Renal papillary necrosis. In both kidneys the renal papillae show greyish necrosis; on the right, some of the papillae have sloughed off. Renal papillary necrosis most often occurs as a complication of diabetes mellitus, analgesic abuse, sickle cell anaemia or urinary obstruction with superadded infection. Microvascular damage is thought to be responsible in most cases; renal colic or oliguria may result.

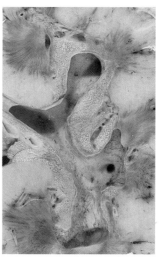

Fig.8.26 Renal amyloidosis. The renal parenchyma shows waxy pallor with blurring of the cortico medullary junction. The kidney is more often involved in secondary than primary or myeloma-associated amyloidosis. Amyloid is a fibrillary protein, arranged in β-pleated sheets, which is derived from serum amyloid A protein in secondary cases and from immunoglobulin light chains in the primary or myeloma-associated group. Renal involvement is bilateral and usually results in proteinuria and chronic renal failure.

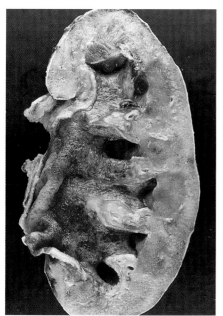

Fig.8.25 Hydro-nephrosis. The pelvicalyceal system is grossly dilated, with marked atrophy of the cortex and medulla. There is florid pyelitis. Hydronephrosis results from distal urinary obstruction, causes of which include prostatic enlargement, pelvic or ureteric tumours, ureteric calculi, neuromuscular defects and retro-peritoneal fibrosis. This condition is often complicated by urinary infection but renal function is impaired only if the obstruction is bilateral.

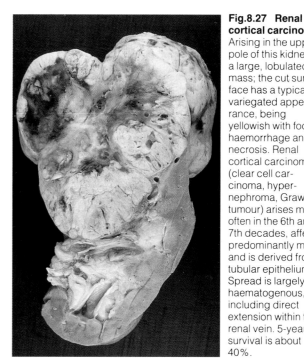

Fig.8.27 Renal cortical carcinoma. Arising in the upper pole of this kidney is a large, lobulated mass; the cut surface has a typically variegated appearance, being yellowish with foci of haemorrhage and necrosis. Renal cortical carcinoma (clear cell carcinoma, hypernephroma, Grawitz tumour) arises most often in the 6th and 7th decades, affects predominantly men and is derived from tubular epithelium. Spread is largely haematogenous, including direct extension within the renal vein. 5-year-survival is about 40%.

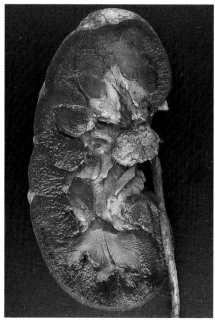

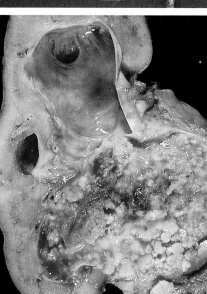

Fig.8.28 Pelvic transitional cell carcinoma (TCC). Above, a small papillary tumour is seen arising in the renal pelvis; below, a much larger, more solid tumour has filled the renal pelvis and caused secondary hydro-nephrosis. TCC of the renal pelvis is not uncommon, arises most often in the 6th and 7th decades and may be associated with similar lesions in the bladder or ureter. Workers in the aniline dye and rubber industries, along with cigarette smokers, are at increased risk. Overall 5-year-survival is about 40%, solid tumours carrying a worse prognosis than papillary. The development of multifocal neo-plasms along the length of the urinary tract is now regarded as a 'field-change' effect rather than metastatic 'seeding' from a proximal lesion.

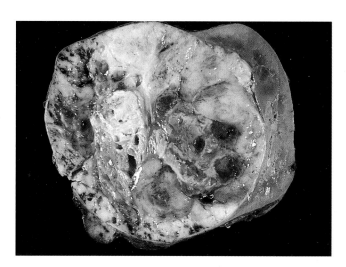

Fig.8.29 Nephroblastoma. This kidney is largely replaced by a large, well circumscribed tumour. The cut surface is pale with cystic, haemorrhagic and myxoid foci. Nephroblastoma (Wilm's tumour) is one of the commonest malignancies in infancy, affects predominantly males and almost invariably presents by the age of 7 years. It may occasionally be bilateral or associated with corporal hemihyper-trophy or aniridia. With modern multimodal therapy, the prognosis is extremely good.

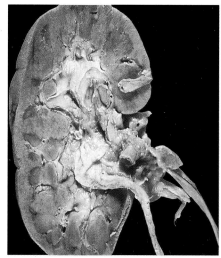

Fig.8.30 Ureteric duplication. Ema-nating from this renal pelvis are two separate ureters. The kidney is other-wise normal. Congenital anomalies of the urinary tract are common and may be associated with genital tract malfor-mations. Up to 3% of the population may have accessory ureters, although the bifurcation is usually distal to the renal pelvis.

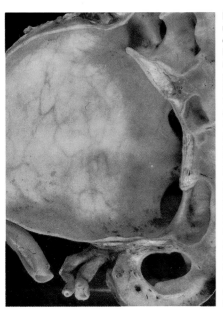

Fig.8.31 Pelvi-ureteric junction obstruction. This kidney shows marked hydronephrosis with gross pelvic dilatation. *In vivo*, two aberrant arteries (bottom right) were compressing the proximal end of the ureter (bottom left). Obstruction at the pelvi-ureteric junction is an important cause of hydronephrosis and may be due to idiopathic neuromuscular incoordination or a developmental anomaly of the renal vessels or ureter.

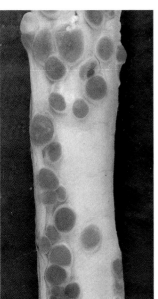

Fig.8.32 Ureteritis cystica. Projecting from the urothelial surface of the ureter are multiple, small, thin-walled, cystic structures. Ureteritis cystica represents a result of long-standing chronic inflammation, of whatever cause, and is entirely comparable to cystitis cystica in the bladder. The cysts are dilated von Brunn's nests, which are localised downgrowths of urothelium often seen in chronic inflammation. Occasionally ureteritis cystica may give rise to ureteric obstruction.

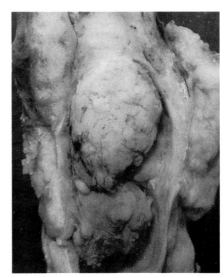

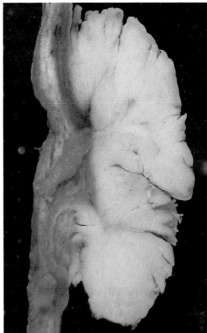

Fig.8.33 Ureteric transitional cell carcinoma (TCC). Emanating from the posterior wall of this thickened ureter is a rounded solid tumour (top); a cross-section through a separate lesion demonstrates well the typical papillary nature of a TCC (bottom). The pathology of ureteric TCC is much the same as that in the renal pelvis (see Fig.8.28). Multifocal TCC in the urinary tract is common, and is thought to represent a 'field-change' effect. It is said that the thinness of the ureteric wall predisposes to early deep invasion of these tumours and hence to rapid lymphatic spread. Generally, the prognosis of these tumours is worse than that of their counterparts in the bladder.

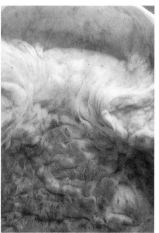

Fig.8.34 Bladder diverticulum. Projecting from the fundus of the bladder is a thin-walled diverticular sac (above); the bladder itself is trabeculated and markedly congested. Bladder diverticula are usually a consequence of outflow tract obstruction and are therefore commonest in elderly males with prostatic hypertrophy. Because urine stagnates within such diverticula, secondary infection and stone formation are common. The development of carcinoma is also a well recognised complication.

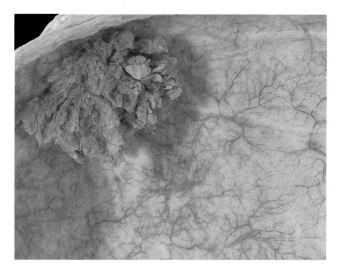

Fig.8.35 Vesical papillary transitional cell carcinoma (TCC). Projecting from the urothelial surface is a small papillary tumour composed of innumerable frond-like excrescences. In the urinary tract, the bladder is the commonest site of origin of TCC. In addition to the aetiological factors mentioned in Fig.8.28, other predisposing causes include schistosomiasis, bladder diverticula and exstrophy. Multifocality is common and the overall mortality is about 50%, many deaths resulting from the complications of obstruction or infection rather than from metastases.

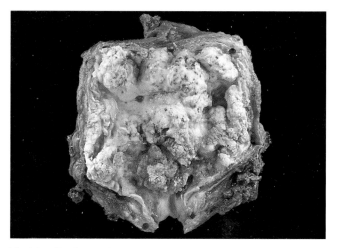

Fig.8.36 Vesical solid transitional cell carcinoma (TCC). This bladder has been opened to show gross urothelial distortion by a multilobulated, predominantly solid, pale neoplasm. A papillary area is visible just above the urethral orifice. Solid vesical TCC is less common than the papillary variant, although the two patterns may be mixed. Solid lesions, which are usually poorly differentiated histologically, carry a worse prognosis.

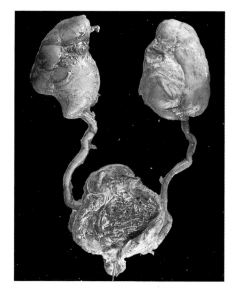

Fig.8.37 Urethral valve. A flap of redundant epithelium is visible in the prostatic urethra (marked with a green probe); the bladder is trabeculated and congested and there is marked bilateral hydroureter and hydronephrosis. This congenital malformation is virtually confined to males and is one of the commonest causes of urinary obstruction in infancy. Age at presentation is dependent upon the degree of obstruction.

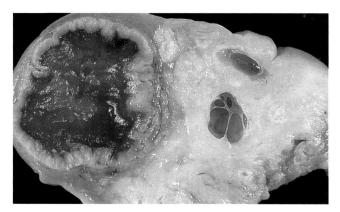

Fig.9.1 Corpus luteum. Within the ovary is a well circumscribed nodule, measuring 1.5 cm in diameter. The outer rim is bright yellow in colour, while centrally it is composed of loose haemorrhagic tissue within which is a small cavity. The ovarian follicle transforms into a corpus luteum after ovulation, during the course of which haemorrhage into the central cavity is invariable. The yellow rim represents the luteinised granulosa and theca cell layers, which at this stage secrete progesterone and, to a lesser extent, oestrogen in preparation for implantation. If fertilisation does not occur, the corpus luteum involutes.

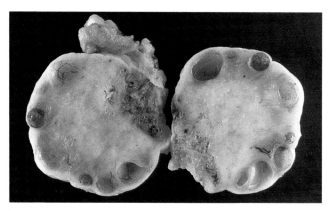

Fig.9.3 Cystic follicles. This bisected ovary shows several small, smooth-walled cystic spaces beneath the serosal surface. Such cysts represent germinal follicles which have undergone partial maturation, but then become atretic and cystic rather than rupturing. They are a common finding in perimenopausal women, in whom deteriorating ovarian function may be contributory. Occasionally they are associated with continued oestrogen secretion and thus may cause endometrial hyperplasia (see Fig.9.30). Larger examples may be described as follicular cysts.

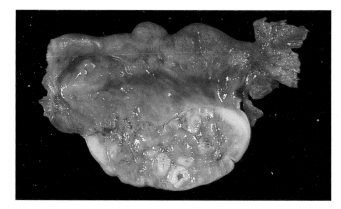

Fig.9.2 Corpora albicantia. This atrophic ovary from an elderly woman contains multiple small, yellowish-white nodules. Corpora albicantia represent corpora lutea which have undergone physiological involution, being replaced largely by hyalinised collagen: as such, they persist after the menopause when they become unduly conspicuous as a consequence of ovarian atrophy.

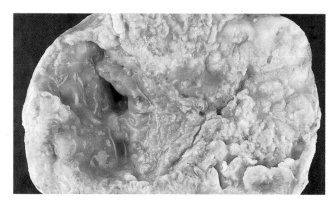

Fig.9.4 Tubo-ovarian abscess. The ovary and adherent fallopian tube (left) show extensive suppuration and haemorrhage. Such pyogenic oophoritis is most often associated with acute salpingitis (see Fig.9.22), but may occasionally result from haematogenous spread of infection from elsewhere. An important cause of infective oophoritis, although non-pyogenic, is mumps, which may impair fertility. Susprisingly, tuberculous salpingitis only rarely spreads to involve the ovary.

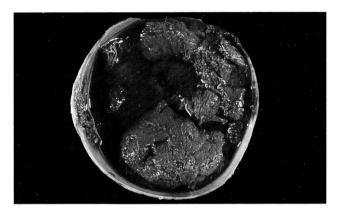

Fig.9.5 Ovarian endometriosis ('chocolate' cyst). The bulk of this ovary is replaced by a haemorrhagic cystic cavity, filled with blood clot. Endometriosis (i.e. ectopic endometrial tissue outside the uterus) is commonest in the ovary, broad ligament and pouch of Douglas but may be seen almost anywhere. The aetiology is uncertain, but the ectopic endometrium undergoes normal cyclical changes, including menstrual bleeding which results in the formation of a 'chocolate' cyst. Interestingly, this condition is often cured by pregnancy.

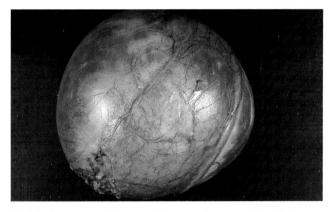

Fig.9.6 Serous cystadenoma. The ovary is replaced by a thin-walled, fairly large unilocular cyst, over the surface of which the fallopian tube is stretched (bottom right). Serous cystadenomas are the commonest benign ovarian neoplasms and are derived from surface epithelium. They are typically smaller than their mucinous counterparts, are bilateral in up to 30% of cases and often show papillary excrescences on the internal surface.

CLASSIFICATION OF OVARIAN TUMOURS

EPITHELIAL	Serous cystadenoma/carcinoma
	Mucinous cystadenoma/carcinoma
	Endometrioid carcinoma
	Mesonephroid adenofibroma/carcinoma
	Brenner tumour
SEX-CORD STROMAL	Granulosa cell tumour
	Thecoma
	Hilar cell tumour (arrhenoblastoma)
GERM CELL	Teratoma
	Dysgerminoma
	Choriocarcinoma
STROMAL MESENCHYME	Fibroma/sarcoma
	Leiomyoma/sarcoma
	Lipoma/sarcoma
UNCERTAIN HISTOGENESIS	Yolk sac tumour
MISCELLANEOUS	Secondary carcinoma
	Lymphoma primary secondary

Fig.9.7 Classification of ovarian tumours.

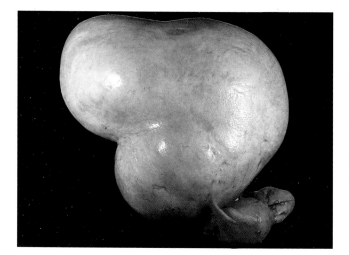

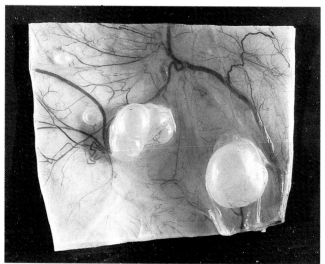

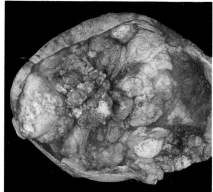

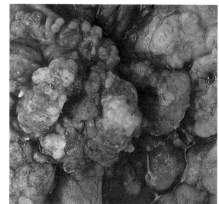

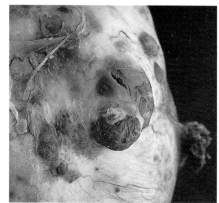

Fig.9.9 Serous cystadeno-carcinoma. The ovary is replaced by a large unilocular tumour (top), the lining of which (middle) is composed of solid, papillary tumour showing haemorrhage and focal necrosis. Below, in a different example, tumour can be seen extending through the serosal surface. Serous cystadeno-carcinoma is the commonest primary ovarian malignancy and is bilateral in up to 40% of cases. Women in the 6th and 7th decades are most often affected and 5-year-survival is only of the order of 25%. It is important to note that a group of serous and mucinous tumours of borderline malignancy can be defined histologically; these carry a much better prognosis.

Fig.9.8 Mucinous cystadenoma. Replacing the ovary is a very large, multiloculated, smooth cyst (top); the uterine fundus is visible in the bottom right-hand corner for size comparison. Below, a portion of this cyst's lining shows multiple, small locules filled with glairy fluid. Mucinous cystadenomas are common benign tumours, derived from ovarian surface epithelium. They arise most often in the 3rd and 4th decades, are bilateral in 10% of cases and may attain an enormous size. Rupture or leakage may give rise to pseudomyxoma peritonei.

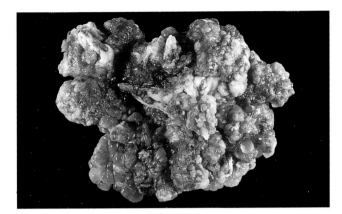

Fig.9.10 Mucinous cystadenocarcinoma. The ovary is replaced by a solid, haemorrhagic mass composed of multiple papillae and locules, containing viscid fluid. Mucinous cystadenocarcinoma is common, arising largely in the middle-aged or elderly and, like its benign counterpart, may attain a great size. It is derived from ovarian surface epithelium, as is its serous equivalent, but carries a better prognosis, with a 5-year-survival rate of up to 50%.

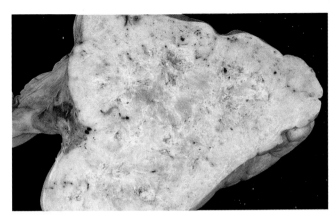

Fig.9.12 Brenner tumour. The ovary is replaced by a well circumscribed, irregular neoplasm, the cut surface of which is yellowish-white with mucoid and fibrous foci. Brenner tumours are derived from ovarian surface epithelium but show Wolffian differentiation. They are comparatively uncommon but may arise at any age and are sometimes bilateral. In the vast majority of cases these tumours are benign.

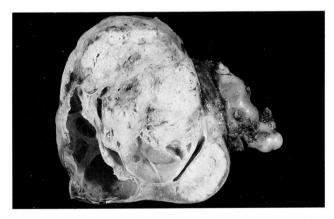

Fig.9.11 Mesonephroid adenocarcinoma. Arising in the ovary is a large, predominantly solid, yellowish neoplasm which shows focal cystic change and necrosis. Mesonephroid (clear cell) adeno-carcinoma is uncommon and is also derived from ovarian surface epithelium (despite its mistaken nomenclature). The clinical features are almost exactly the same as those of serous cystadenocarcinoma (see Fig. 9.9).

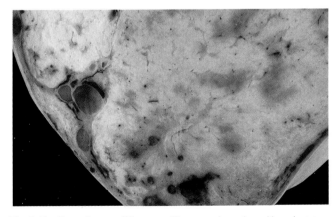

Fig.9.13 Granulosa cell tumour. The ovary is replaced by a large, well circumscribed, yellow tumour, within which are small foci of cystic change. Granulosa cell tumours, which are sex-cord stromal in origin, are relatively uncommon but arise most often in the peri-menopausal years. They should be regarded as malignant (although often low-grade) and they typically secrete excessive oestrogens, leading to endometrial hyperplasia or carcinoma. Rare cases seen in young girls usually give rise to precocious pseudopuberty.

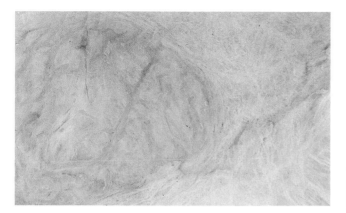

Fig.9.14 Thecoma. The cut surface of this small ovarian tumour is predominantly fibrous but shows a typical area of yellowish colouration, representing accumulated lipid. Thecomas are sex-cord stromal tumours which most often arise perimenopausally. While they are almost invariably benign, they commonly secrete excessive oestrogens which may result in the development of endometrial hyperplasia or carcinoma.

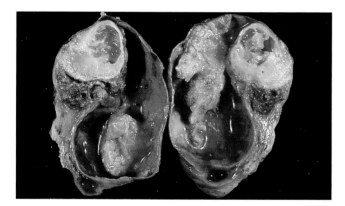

Fig.9.15 Mature cystic teratoma. The ovary has been bisected to show replacement by a multicystic tumour, within which sebaceous material and matted hair are evident. Mature cystic teratoma (or benign ovarian dermoid) is a common germ cell tumour which arises most often in the 2nd to 4th decades. It is particularly prone to undergoing torsion (see Fig.9.19), often being pedunculated. Struma ovarii is an uncommon variant of the same tumour, composed predominantly of thyroid tissue. Malignant ovarian teratomas are very uncommon (cf. testicular teratomas).

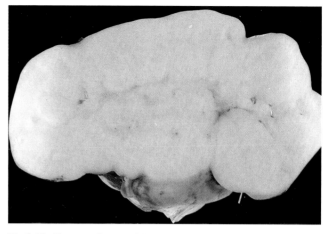

Fig.9.16 Dysgerminoma. Arising in this ovary is a large, uniform, well circumscribed, whitish tumour, similar in appearance to a potato. Dysgerminomas are comparatively uncommon germ cell tumours which show no identifiable differentiation. They are commonest between 10 and 30 years, are analogous to the testicular seminoma (see Fig.10.3) and should be regarded as malignant. They are extremely radiosensitive and the prognosis is excellent.

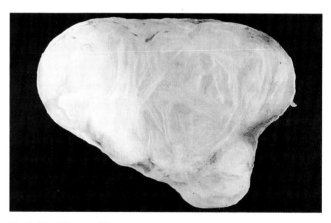

Fig.9.17 Fibroma. The ovary is replaced by a pale, lobulated tumour, the cut surface of which is fibrous and whorled. Ovarian fibromas are derived from stromal mesenchyme, usually arise in the 5th and 6th decades and are almost invariably benign. They may be associated with the development of ascites or pleural effusions (Meigs' syndrome), an entirely unexplained phenomenon.

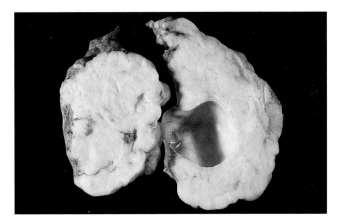

Fig.9.18 Metastasis to the ovary. Both ovaries are diffusely replaced by pale, rather nodular tumour, in this case of breast origin. Note also the follicular cyst (right). The ovary is not infrequently the site of metastasis, particularly from primary carcinomas of the endometrium, gastro-intestinal tract and breast. Bilateral involvement is common. The term Krukenberg tumour is reserved *only* for those metastases, (most often of gastric origin) which histologically show a signet-ring, mucus-secreting pattern.

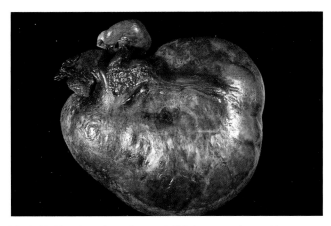

Fig.9.19 Torsion of ovarian cyst. This large ovarian cyst has twisted about the fallopian tube and broad ligament (top) resulting in tense, haemorrhagic engorgement. Ovarian torsion is not uncommon in association with an ovarian cyst or neoplasm, the size or weight of which results in twisting of the broad ligament or mesovarium. Peritonitis or gangrene may rapidly develop.

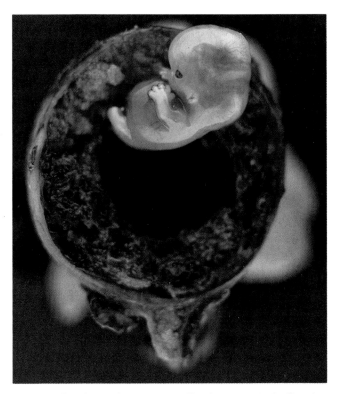

Fig.9.20 Tubal ectopic pregnancy. This fallopian tube is dilated and the wall is thickened and haemorrhagic; within the lumen lies a tiny 9 week fetus. Ectopic implantation of the fertilised ovum is commonest in the fallopian tube, most often in its ampullary portion. About 1 in 100 pregnancies are ectopic; possible causes include previous tubal inflammation or impaired tubal motility. Up to 60% of tubal ectopics rupture, usually by about the 12th week.

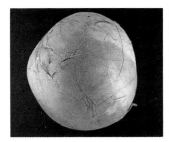

Fig.9.21 Paratubal cyst. This is a simple, smooth-walled, fluid-filled cyst which was an incidental finding in the broad ligament. Such cysts are insignificant benign structures which may be derived from the ovarian hilum or from vestiges of the mesonephric (Wolffian), paramesonephric (Müllerian) or Gartner's ducts.

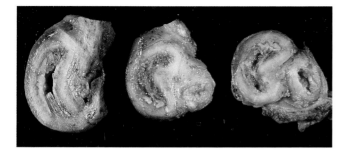

Fig.9.22 Acute salpingitis. Serial sections through this fallopian tube show florid luminal suppuration and congestion. Acute salpingitis is most often sexually transmitted: the most frequent organisms responsible are chlamydia, mycoplasma or anaerobes. The gonococcus is now thought to be only an initiating factor. Other predisposing factors include abortion, surgical instrumentation and the use of an intra-uterine contraceptive device.

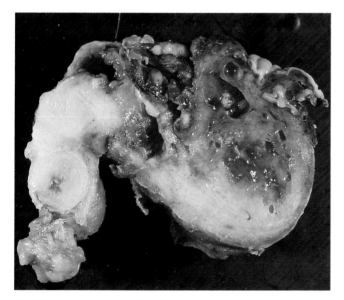

Fig.9.23 Chronic salpingitis. While the lumen of this fallopian tube is focally patent (left), the remainder is distorted by a fibrotic and focally necrotic mass. In such cases, it is uncommon to isolate the infective organism but tubal damage such as this is frequently bilateral and may result in infertility. Macroscopically, tuberculous salpingitis may look very similar.

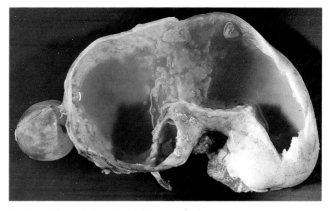

Fig.9.24 Pyosalpinx. This fallopian tube is grossly dilated and distorted and the lumen contains yellowish, purulent debris. Note also the simple paratubal cyst (left). This appearance is another possible outcome of chronic salpingitis but may also be seen in very severe acute infection. Bilateral involvement is again common.

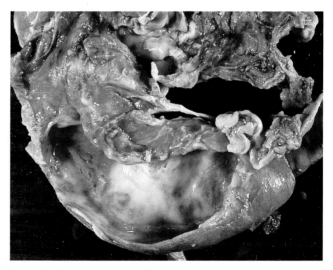

Fig.9.25 Hydrosalpinx. This fallopian tube is dilated and rather elongated and the lumen contains milky, clear fluid. Note the dense adhesions to paratubal structures. This appearance, which is seen in the ampullary portion of the tube, is most often due to long-standing, low-grade infection but may also be associated with idiopathic pelvic inflammatory disease.

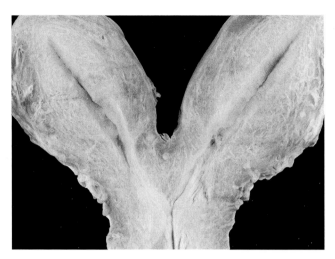

Fig.9.26 Bicornuate uterus. This specimen shows two apparently normal uterine cavities which converge on a single cervical canal. This is a congenital malformation, representing partial failure of fusion of the Müllerian ducts. Up to 1 in 500 women have developmental anomalies of varying severity in the genital tract, which may give rise to menstrual or obstetric problems.

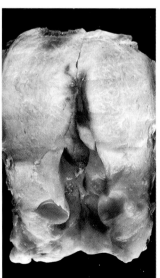

Fig.9.27 Endometrial polyp and Nabothian cysts. This coronal section of the uterus shows a polypoid lesion arising from the endometrium: in addition there are several smooth cystic cavities in the endocervix. Endometrial polyps are common, most often peri-menopausal, lesions which may be multiple. Whether they represent true benign neo-plasms or a localised reaction to oestrogen hypersensitivity is uncertain. Nabothian cysts represent cystic dilation of endocervical glands and are of no known significance.

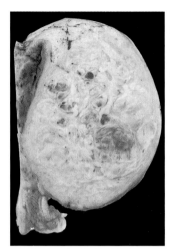

Fig.9.28 Localised adenomyosis. This sagittal section through a uterus shows a well circumscribed, whorled mass in the anterior wall, within which there are haemorrhagic and yellowish areas. Adenomyosis is defined as the presence of endometrium deep in the myometrium and is commonest in parous peri-menopausal women. It results from downward extension of the basal endometrium and either involves the uterus diffusely or is localised, as here, when it may be known as an 'adenomyoma'. The aetiology is possibly related to excessive oestrogenic stimulation.

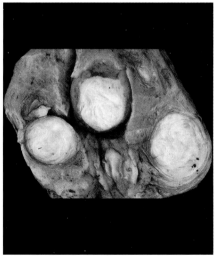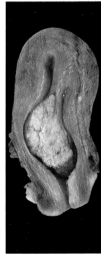

Fig.9.29 Uterine leiomyomata. The uterus on the left shows several well circumscribed, whorled fibrous neoplasms within the myometrium; that on the right shows a single, pedunculated sub-mucosal tumour of a similar nature which is distorting the endometrial cavity. Uterine leiomyomata ('fibroids') are very common benign tumours of smooth muscle which develop during the reproductive years, probably as a result of oestrogen sensitivity. Degenerative changes, including calcification or infarction, are common.

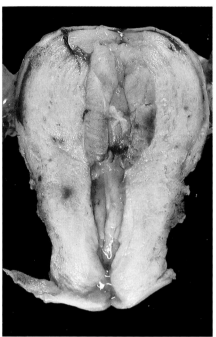

Fig.9.30 Endometrial hyperplasia. Within the body of the uterus, the endometrial lining shows irregular, almost polypoid thickening. Endometrial hyperplasia, which is associated with cystic dilatation of endometrial glands, is due to unopposed oestrogen stimulation as may occur in anovulatory menstrual cycles or in association with ovarian sex-cord stromal tumours. Histologically atypical variants of this condition may be associated with the development of endometrial adenocarcinoma.

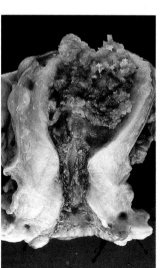

Fig.9.31 Endometrial adenocarcinoma. Arising from the endometrium in the body of the uterus is a large, polypoid, focally necrotic neoplasm. Endometrial carcinoma is not uncommon and occurs most often after the menopause. Proven associations include nulliparity, infertility and obesity, all of which are thought to be co-factors of excessive oestrogen stimulation. The 5-year-survival rate is of the order of 70%, dependent upon histological grade and staging.

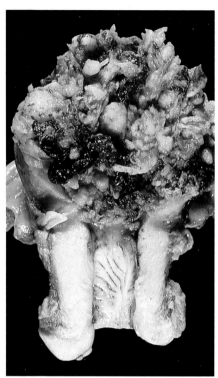

Fig.9.32 Malignant mixed Müllerian tumour. Arising in the uterine fundus is a large, polypoid, haemorrhagic mass. Extensive myometrial invasion is apparent. Malignant mixed Müllerian tumours are derived from Müllerian mesenchyme and thus contain both epithelial and connective tissue elements. They arise most often in the elderly and carry a poor prognosis. Mixed Müllerian tumours may sometimes have only one malignant component, which is usually mesenchymal, (adenosarcoma) or be entirely benign (adenofibroma).

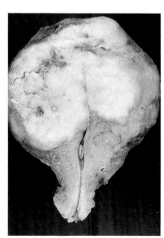

Fig.9.33 Uterine leiomyosarcoma. In the myometrium of the fundus and body is an irregular, pale neoplasm showing focal haemorrhage and necrosis. Serosal invasion is apparent (top). Leiomyosarcoma of the uterus is comparatively rare, usually occurs in the 5th and 6th decades and may be associated with nulliparity. These tumours arise de novo and not from leiomyomas: the 5-year-survival is about 30%.

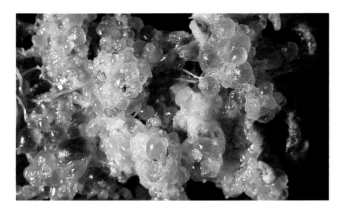

Fig.9.34 Hydatidiform mole. This specimen consists of a mass of grape-like hydropic villi which has been removed from the uterine cavity. Hydatidiform mole arises in about 1 in 1,500 U.K. pregnancies but is much commoner in the Far East. Such moles are derived from abnormal trophoblastic proliferation and usually affect females at the extremes of reproductive life. Up to 3% go on to develop choriocarcinoma and therefore careful follow-up by serum β-HCG estimations is mandatory.

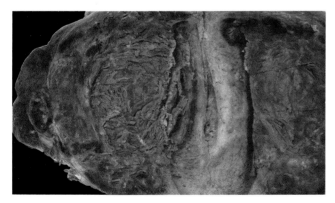

Fig.9.35 Choriocarcinoma. This uterus has been opened to show diffuse replacement of the myometrium by an extensive haemorrhagic tumour. Choriocarcinoma is a malignant tumour of trophoblast, the incidence of which parallels that of hydatidiform mole, since 50% of cases are preceded by a mole. It may also arise following spontaneous abortion or a normal pregnancy. Despite a tendency to extensive vascular invasion, up to 90% of affected patients are cured by chemotherapy in conjunction with careful follow-up using β-HCG estimations.

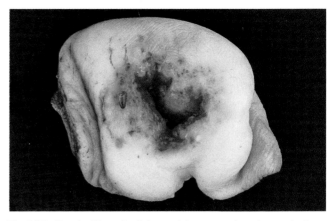

Fig.9.36 Cervical 'erosion'. Around the external os, the cervical epithelium appears reddish. This appearance is, in fact, physiological and is not due to epithelial erosion at all. Rather, it is due to eversion of endocervical mucosa, which occurs with elongation of the endocervical canal during adolescence, and which then undergoes squamous metaplasia.

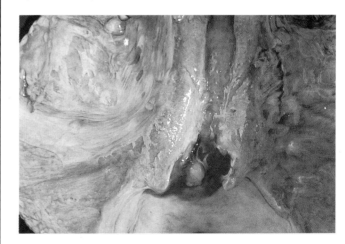

Fig.9.37 Endocervical polyp. A close-up view of the endocervical canal and vaginal vault shows a small, rather mucoid polyp in the endocervical canal, surrounded by operative haemorrhage. Endocervical polyps are extremely common, occurring most often in the 4th and 5th decades, and represent focal hyperplasia of the endocervical epithelium. Superimposed inflammation is common but malignant change is excessively rare.

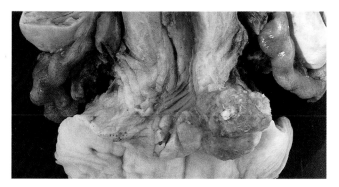

Fig.9.38 Cervical squamous carcinoma. Arising from the ectocervix is an irregular, fungating, pale neoplasm. Carcinoma of the cervix is common and increasing in incidence; while it occurs most frequently in the 5th and 6th decades, younger women are not infrequently affected. It is thought to arise in pre-existent areas of intra-epithelial neoplasia (dysplasia) over a period of 10 to 20 years. Aetiologically, *Herpes simplex* type II and human papillomavirus types 16 and 18 are thought to be important, with early age at first coitus being the most critical co-factor. Overall 5-year-survival is about 50%, dependent upon the degree of invasion.

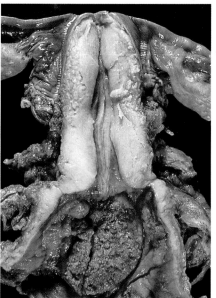

Fig.9.39 Vaginal squamous carcinoma. Arising in the posterior vaginal wall is a raised, irregular neoplasm. Squamous carcinoma of the vagina is a rare tumour of the elderly, which is probably aetio-logically similar to cervical carcinoma. Vaginal adeno-carcinoma is also extremely uncommon but is typically a tumour of young girls, whose mothers were treated with di-ethylstilboestrol during pregnancy.

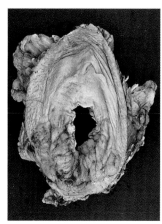

Fig.9.40 Vulval Bowen's disease. This simple vulvectomy specimen shows a raised, rather nodular, reddish area around the inferior margins of the introitus. Vulval Bowen's disease (intra-epithelial neoplasia) represents carcinoma-in-situ and is not uncommon, particularly with increasing age. Aetiologically, the viruses implicated in cervical carcinoma are thought to be important (see Fig.9.38). Progression to invasive carcinoma is not uncommon but occurs most often in the elderly or immunosuppressed.

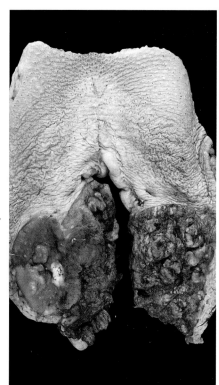

Fig.9.41 Vulval squamous carcinoma. The labia majora of this radical vulvectomy specimen are diffusely infiltrated by a raised, nodular and focally ulcerated neoplasm. Vulval carcinoma occurs most often in the 7th and 8th decades, usually in cases with pre-existent intra-epithelial neoplasia or chronic inflam-mation. Overall 5-year-survival is about 70%. A rare, very well differen-tiated warty variant, known as verrucous carcinoma, only very rarely metastasises and has a better prognosis.

10 Male Reproductive System

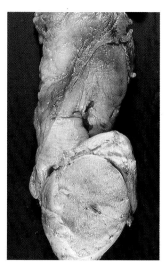

Fig.10.1 Testicular atrophy. A coronal section through this testis shows that it is much smaller than normal, particularly when compared to the spermatic cord (above). Well recognised causes of testicular atrophy include maldescent, oestrogen therapy, alcoholism, irradiation, Klinefelter's syndrome and hormonal abnormalities of the hypothalamic-pituitary-adrenal axis. Such testes typically show markedly diminished or absent spermatogenesis.

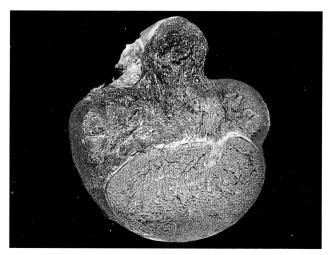

Fig.10.2 Testicular torsion. The testis, epididymis and distal spermatic cord show dark haemorrhagic infarction. This condition is, in fact, due to torsion of the spermatic cord, in which venous obstruction occurs first, resulting in intense distal congestion. It is commonest in the 2nd decade and is usually due to an abnormally long or malorientated spermatic cord or mesorchium. Early diagnosis may allow preservation of testicular function and contralateral orchidopexy should always be performed.

CLASSIFICATION OF TESTICULAR TUMOURS

GERM CELL	Seminoma	classical	38%
		spermatocytic	2%
	Teratoma	differentiated	1%
		intermediate	20%
		undifferentiated	10%
		trophoblastic	1%
	Combined seminoma/ teratoma		14%
NON-GERM CELL	Yolk sac tumour		1%
	Leydig cell tumour		2%
	Sertoli cell tumour		1.5%
OTHER	Lymphoma	primary secondary	7%
	Leukaemic infiltration		<1%
	Metastases		<1%

Fig.10.3 Classification of testicular tumours (modified information from the U.K. Testicular Tumour Panel). These figures represent percentages of the total number of testicular tumours.

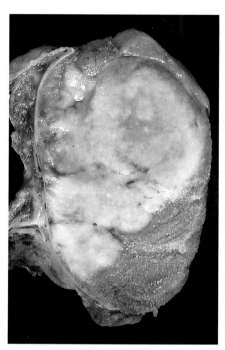

Fig.10.4 Seminoma. Much of this testis is replaced by a well circumscribed, lobulated pinkish-white tumour. Seminomas are the commonest primary testicular tumour and are derived from germinal cells. They occur most often in the 4th decade and are the most frequent tumours to arise in an un-descended testis. They are indistin-guishable from the female ovarian dysgerminoma (see Fig.9.16). Seminomas are extremely radio-sensitive and 5-year-survival is now at least 90%.

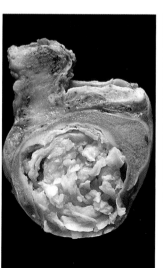

Fig.10.5 Differentiated teratoma. Within this testis is a well circumscribed mass which is multicystic and contains yellowish keratinous debris. Differentiated teratomas are uncommon, accounting for only about 2% of testicular teratomas, and may arise at any age from birth to 30 years. They are composed solely of mature tissue from any of the three germinal layers but, despite their apparently benign nature, up to 10% metastasise, particularly those occurring in young adults.

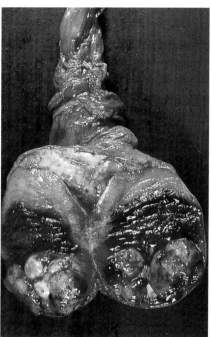

Fig.10.6 Malignant teratoma inter-mediate (MTI). The lower pole of the testis is replaced by a multinodular, rather necrotic tumour, above which is an extensive zone of infarction due to torsion. MTI, which retains some differentiated foci (in contrast to MTU) is typically a tumour of young adult males. It tends to both haematogenous and lymphatic spread and the 5-year-survival is about 55% (better than MTU or MTT). Note that any testicular tumour may predi-spose to, and occasionally present with, torsion.

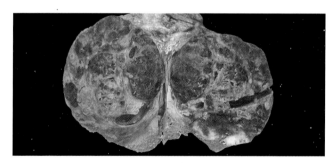

Fig.10.7 Malignant teratoma trophoblastic (MTT). This testis is completely replaced by a multinodular, dark, haemorrhagic mass showing paler foci of necrosis. MTT (or choriocarcinoma) is the rarest subtype of teratoma and is typified by the presence of syncytio-trophoblast and cytotrophoblast. Characteristically this tumour is very haemorrhagic. The prognosis was previously abysmal, but the use of both modern multimodal therapy and β-human chorionic gonadotrophin as a serum marker has led to greatly improved survival.

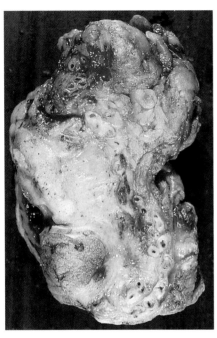

Fig.10.8 Chronic epididymitis. The epididymis and distal spermatic cord are markedly thickened and fibrotic and in places, obstructed ducts are visibly dilated. There is secondary testicular atrophy. Epididymitis is usually associated with lower urinary tract infection or urethritis and is commonest in adulthood. The condition is most often unilateral and may spread locally to the testis or tunica vaginalis. Recurrent infection and chronicity are not uncommon.

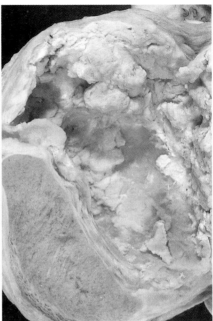

Fig.10.10 Tuberculous epididymitis. The epididymis is totally replaced by an irregular cavity containing copious caseous material. The testis is compressed but completely spared. Tuberculous epididymitis is most often seen in young adults, usually in association with TB of the urinary tract: it has become very uncommon in the indigenous Western population. Bilateral infection is frequent and while the spermatic cord may be affected, the testis is only rarely involved.

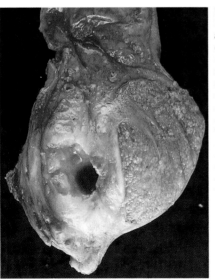

Fig.10.9 Epididymal abscess. The epididymis appears rather thickened and scarred but in addition, there is a small central abscess cavity with adjacent congestion. The testis shows partial atrophy. This is an example of acute-on-chronic infection which, in very severe cases, may be complicated by abscess formation. Gonococci are often isolated from such a lesion.

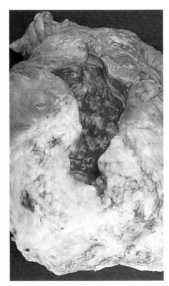

Fig.10.11 Prostatic adenocarcinoma. A transverse section through the whole prostate gland, near the bladder neck, shows diffuse replacement by pale, irregular and focally necrotic tumour. Residual nodular areas of benign tissue are also present. Prostatic carcinoma is very common from the 6th decade onwards but often pursues an unaggressive course. The aetiology may be hormonal. The outer prostatic glands are the usual site of origin, particularly in the posterior lobe. A raised serum level of tartrate-labile acid phosphatase is a useful diagnostic marker and metastasis to bone is a characteristic feature of this tumour.

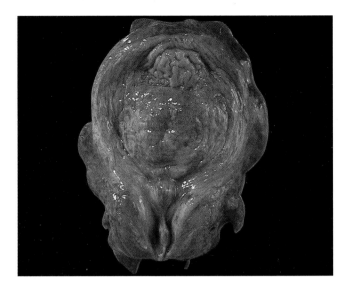

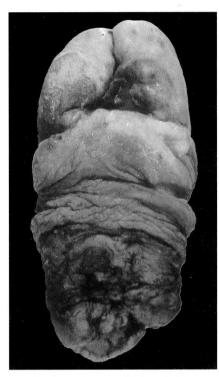

Fig.10.13 Penile squamous carcinoma. Arising at the base of the glans penis (top) is a pale, ulcerating neoplasm, which is better seen in cross-section (bottom). Squamous carcinoma of the penis is relatively uncommon in the Western World, but tends to arise in elderly uncircumcised men. In some cases there may be pre-existent Bowen's disease. The majority of these tumours develop from the glans penis or the prepuce. While this tumour tends to exophytic or locally invasive growth, metastasis is usually a late phenomenon. However, presentation is often delayed by the patient's shyness or mistaken belief that he has a venereal disease.

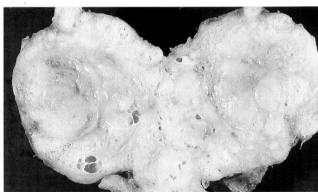

Fig.10.12 Benign prostatic hypertrophy. Above, the prostate and bladder of an elderly male are shown. The prostate is hypertrophied with a particularly prominent median lobe obstructing the bladder neck. The bladder wall is thickened and trabeculated. Below, a transverse section through a retropubic prostatectomy specimen shows marked enlargement, the prostatic tissue being composed of multiple yellowish-white nodules. Benign prostatic hypertrophy (nodular or myoadenomatous hyperplasia) is increasingly common with advancing age, being almost universal by the 9th decade. It is due to an, as yet unclear, imbalance between testosterone and oestrogen. The inner group of prostatic glands are typically affected, leading to urinary obstruction. It does *not* predispose to carcinoma.

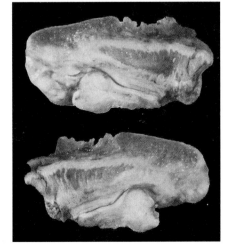

11 Nervous System

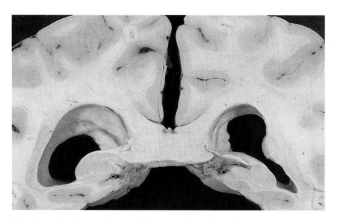

Fig.11.1 Hydrocephalus. This coronal section of brain shows gross dilation of the lateral ventricles, due to obstruction of the cerebral aqueduct by a glioma. Hydrocephalus may be classified into 4 types: *Non-communicating (internal)* due to obstruction of the aqueduct or foramina of the fourth ventricle; *Communicating* due to obstruction at the subarachnoid cisterns; *External* due to impaired reabsorption of CSF; and *Compensatory*, associated with cerebral atrophy.

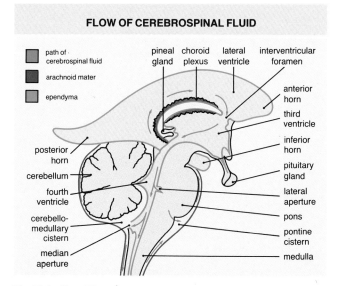

FLOW OF CEREBROSPINAL FLUID

path of cerebrospinal fluid
arachnoid mater
ependyma

pineal gland · choroid plexus · lateral ventricle · interventricular foramen
anterior horn
third ventricle
inferior horn
pituitary gland
lateral aperture
pons
pontine cistern
medulla

posterior horn
cerebellum
fourth ventricle
cerebello-medullary cistern
median aperture

Fig.11.2 Simplified representation of flow of cerebrospinal fluid, seen in the left hemisphere (medial view).

CAUSES OF HYDROCEPHALUS		
CONGENITAL	Arnold-Chiari malformation	
	Bifid aqueduct	
	Atresia of 4th ventricular foramina (Dandy-Walker syndrome)	
	Intra-uterine infection	toxoplasmosis
		syphilis
ACQUIRED	Posterior fossa tumours	
	Post-meningitic	
	Compensatory	

Fig.11.3 Causes of hydrocephalus.

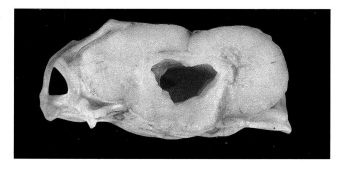

Fig.11.4 Syringomyelia. This segment of cervical spinal cord contains a dilated, cystic cavity (syrinx), which has compressed the central canal anteriorly to a barely discernible slit. Possible associations include fourth ventricle outflow obstruction, resulting in hydromyelia, and neurofibromatosis (see Fig.11.28). Typical clinical features include impaired pain and temperature sensations and the 'claw-hand' deformity, due to nerve tract compression.

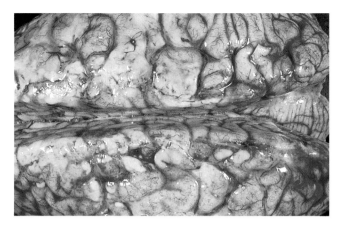

Fig.11.5 Adult bacterial meningitis. The superior surface of the brain is intensely congested and covered in a purulent exudate, particularly over the frontal lobes (left). Suppurative meningitis may complicate endocarditis, middle ear, sinus or pulmonary infections or trauma. Direct spread of organisms may also occur from the nasopharynx. Important pathogenic organisms include *Neisseria meningitidis* (in young children and young adults), *Haemophilus influenzae* in young children and *Streptococcus pneumoniae* in the very young or old. Almost any organism, including fungi, may be responsible in the immunocompromised patient.

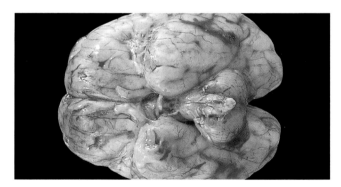

Fig.11.6 Neonatal bacterial meningitis. The surface of this neonate's brain shows congestion and suppuration, especially over the inferior aspect of the right temporal lobe. Neonatal meningitis is seen most often after a prolonged or traumatic delivery and is more common in premature infants. The culpable organism is always derived from the maternal genital tract at birth, most often being *Streptococcus pyogenes* or a coliform, particularly *E. coli*.

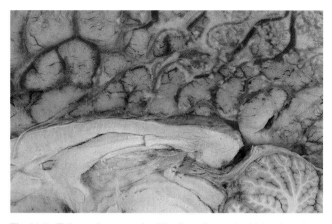

Fig.11.7 Tuberculous meningitis. Over the parietal lobe there is a dense inflammatory exudate associated with numerous adjacent 'tubercles'. Tuberculous meningitis is usually seen as a complication of primary infection in young individuals and is most often due to miliary spread. It may also result from rupture of a localised intra-cerebral tuberculous (Rich) focus into the subarachnoid space. The base of the brain and upper cerebellum are most often affected.

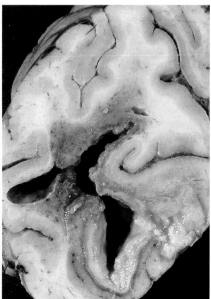

Fig.11.8 Cerebral abscess. Within this left cerebral hemi-sphere is an irregular abscess cavity which is partly walled off. There is surrounding con-gestion. Predi-sposing causes are much the same as those for suppura-tive meningitis (see Fig.11.5), including haematogenous spread of any sys-temic infection. The latter typically leads to abscesses localised in the distribution of the middle cerebral artery.

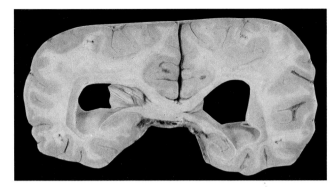

Fig.11.9 General paresis of the insane. This coronal section of brain shows marked cortical atrophy, flattening of the gyral pattern and compensatory hydrocephalus. General paresis is a late (quaternary) manifestation of syphilis. Other macroscopical features include leptomeningeal thickening and granular ependymitis. The resultant neuronal loss may be associated with dementia, epilepsy, motor dysfunction and the Argyll Robertson pupil. Cord involvement in quaternary syphilis gives rise to tabes dorsalis.

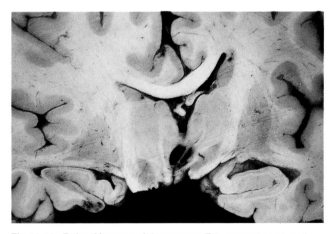

Fig.11.10 Raised intracranial pressure. This coronal section of brain shows marked compression and asymmetry of the left lateral ventricle and, just above, herniation of the cingulate gyrus. Raised intracranial pressure is most often seen in association with intra- or extracerebral haemorrhage, a tumour or extensive infarction. The cardinal macroscopic features, other than those shown here, are tentorial or tonsillar herniation (cerebellar coning) and uncal grooving.

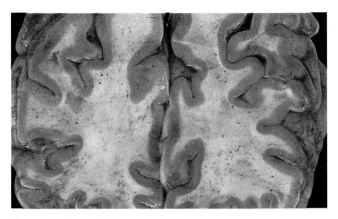

Fig.11.11 Cerebral fat embolism. This section of brain shows numerous small petechial haemorrhages, most notably in the white matter. Fat embolism most commonly results from damage to a major bone, particularly a fracture, in which medullary fat enters the venous system. This may pass unnoticed or may result in impaired cerebral, pulmonary and renal function. Other causes of such haemorrhages include malaria, leukaemia and thrombocytopenic purpura.

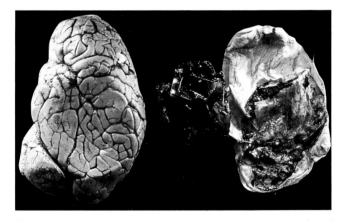

Fig.11.12 Acute subdural haemorrhage. The specimen consists of dura (right), blood clot and the left cerebral hemisphere. An extensive depression is visible in the left temporoparietal region. Subdural haemorrhage is usually traumatic in origin and results from tearing of thin-walled veins as they enter the dural sinuses. Acute lesions may be rapidly fatal if not surgically evacuated, while undetected haemorrhage may result in gradual, chronic cerebral damage.

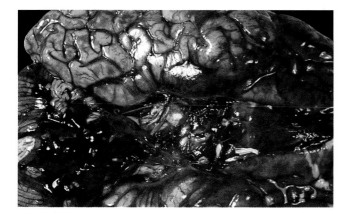

Fig.11.13 Subarachnoid haemorrhage. Rupture of a berry aneurysm of the left posterior cerebral artery has resulted in massive subarachnoid haemorrhage around the base of the brain. Hypertensive rupture of berry aneurysms (see Fig. 11.14) is the commonest source of subarachnoid bleeding but other important causes include trauma and extension of an intracerebral haemorrhage. The prognosis is generally poor.

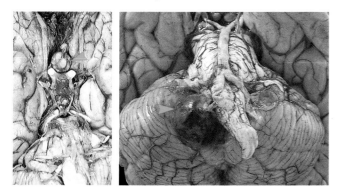

Fig.11.14 Cerebral artery aneurysms. On the left, the frontal lobes have been separated to display a berry aneurysm (arrowed) arising at the junction of the left anterior cerebral and anterior communicating arteries. On the right, an atheromatous saccular aneurysm (see Chapter 1) is seen in the left posterior cerebral artery (arrowed). Berry aneurysms usually result from degenerative changes at the site of a congenital defect in the arterial wall. They may be multiple and are sometimes associated with polycystic renal disease. Other than subarachnoid haemorrhage, they may also be complicated by intracerebral haemorrhage or infarction.

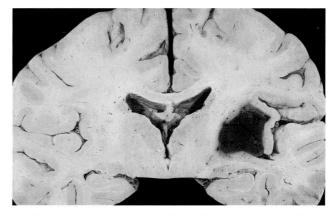

Fig.11.15 Intracerebral haemorrhage. This coronal section of brain shows a recent haemorrhage in the region of the right lentiform nucleus. Intracerebral haemorrhage is less frequently responsible for a 'stroke' (CVA) than cerebral infarction (see Fig.11.17) due to generally better control of essential hypertension. Rupture of Charcot-Bouchard microaneurysms is the commonest cause, although haemorrhage into a neoplasm or abscess is occasionally responsible.

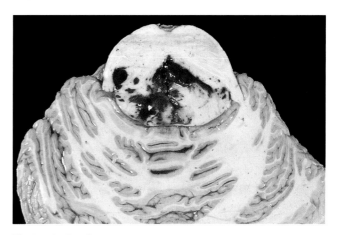

Fig.11.16 Pontine haemorrhage. This section through the pons and cerebellum shows a recent pontine haemorrhage. While this is usually a primary phenomenon (see Fig.11.15), a similar appearance may be seen due to extension of a massive intracortical haemorrhage or compromise of the brain-stem circulation due to tentorial herniation.

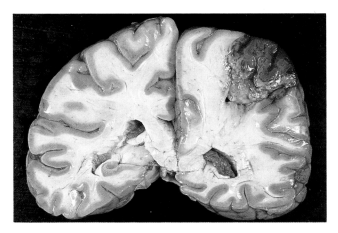

Fig.11.17 Recent cerebral infarct. There is an extensive area of haemorrhagic infarction with a hyperaemic border in the parietal region. Note also the adjacent marked cerebral oedema. Cerebral infarction is the commonest cause of a 'stroke' (CVA) and is most often due to thrombosis in an atheromatous vessel. It may also be embolic in origin (e.g. from the left atrium in atrial fibrillation) or associated with hypercoagulability or the contraceptive pill.

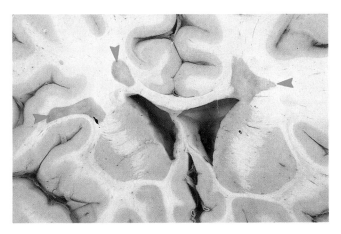

Fig.11.19 Multiple sclerosis. In the periventricular white matter and adjacent internal capsule (left) there are three well-defined grey plaques (arrowed) indicative of foci of demyelination and gliosis. Multiple sclerosis typically affects young adults, particularly females and is a chronic, relapsing and debilitating disease. Aetiologically, a slow viral infection is thought (but not proven) to be responsible, perhaps in combination with genetic factors.

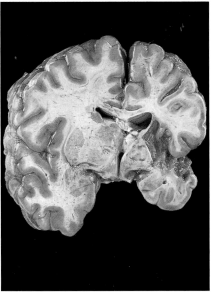

Fig.11.18 Old cerebral infarct. This coronal section of brain shows a massive previous right-sided infarct which has resulted in loss of cortical tissue, cystic degeneration and compensatory hydrocephalus. Multiple (usually small) infarcts over a variable period of time may lead to numerous foci of cerebral softening (status spongiosus) and the clinical syndrome of multi-infarct dementia.

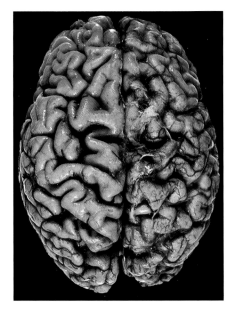

Fig.11.20 Alzheimer's disease. The meninges have been stripped from the left side of this brain to show marked cerebral atrophy, manifest by sulcal widening and diminution of the gyri. Alzheimer's disease is a chronic form of pre-senile dementia, is commonest in the 5th and 6th decades and may also be seen in Down's syndrome. The aetiology is entirely unknown.

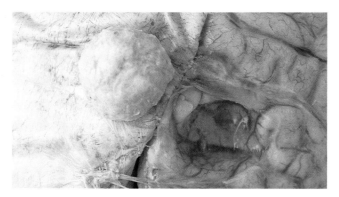

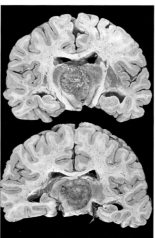

Fig.11.23 Glioblastoma multiforme. These coronal sections of brain show a massive haemorrhagic tumour arising in the basal ganglia and distorting the lateral ventricles. Glioblastoma multiforme is an undifferentiated glial tumour, most often of astrocytic derivation, and occurs predominantly in the 4th and 5th decades. It is the commonest variant of glioma, arises most often in the frontal lobes, septum pellucidum and basal ganglia and carries a very poor prognosis.

Fig.11.21 Meningioma. A circumscribed nodular tumour arising from the meninges (left) has been 'shelled out' of the left parietal lobe, leaving a deep spherical depression. Meningiomas, derived from the arachnoid villi, most often arise in relation to the major venous sinuses. They are slow-growing, almost invariably benign, tumours but may occasionally invade the adjacent skull. They occur predominantly in the 5th and 6th decades and symptoms, if any, depend upon the site of the tumour.

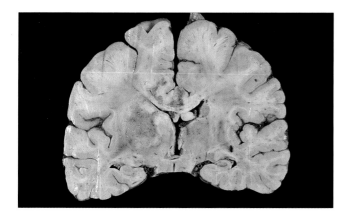

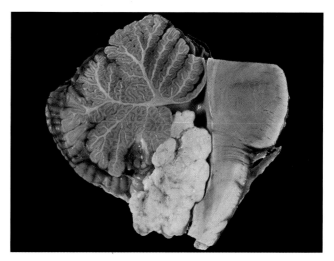

Fig.11.22 Glioma. This coronal section of brain shows an ill-defined neoplasm, with foci of haemorrhage and necrosis in the left hemisphere. There is adjacent oedema and distortion of the ventricular system. Gliomas may be divided, in order of frequency, into glioblastoma multiforme (see Fig 11.23), astrocytoma, oligodendroglioma, ependymoma and choroid plexus papilloma. Mixed types are not uncommon. Gliomas do not give rise to systemic metastases but may 'seed' throughout the CNS and cause death by their local effects.

Fig.11.24 Ependymoma. Arising in the 4th ventricle and compressing the cerebellum posteriorly is a large, multilobulated, white tumour. Ependymomas are one of the least frequent forms of glioma but are the commonest to arise in the spinal cord. They are derived from the ependymal cells that line the ventricular system and cord canal. While typically slow-growing, their location often renders them inoperable and the prognosis is poor.

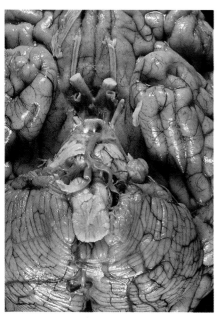

Fig.11.25 Acoustic neuroma. Situated on the left cerebello-pontine angle is a well circumscribed neoplasm arising from the eighth cranial nerve. This is a benign Schwann cell tumour which is sometimes bilateral and may be associated with neurofibromatosis. Clinical features include tinnitus, vertigo and nerve deafness. Complications include compression of other cranial nerves or of the brainstem.

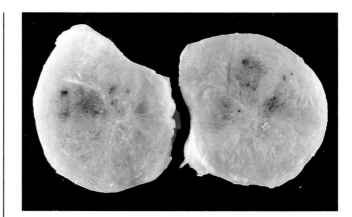

Fig.11.27 Benign schwannoma (neurilemmoma). This is a well circumscribed, encapsulated, small tumour which has a yellowish cut surface and shows small foci of haemorrhage. Benign schwannoma is a common tumour of peripheral nerves and arises from the nerve sheath. It is usually solitary, arises especially in the 3rd to 5th decades and is most often asymptomatic. Occasionally, multiple lesions may be seen in neurofibromatosis but in the latter condition multiple *neurofibromas* are far more common.

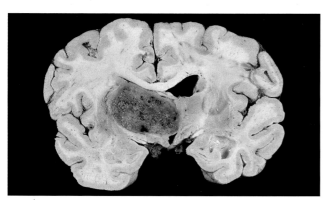

Fig.11.26 Cerebral metastasis. This coronal section of brain shows a solitary, large deposit of focally necrotic and haemorrhagic metastatic tumour, which is situated in the region of the left basal ganglia and is compressing the lateral ventricle. Cerebral metastases, which are usually multiple, are most often situated at the junction of the grey and white matter and are typically well circumscribed (cf. glial tumours). The most frequent primary sites are bronchus, breast, kidney and cutaneous malignant melanoma.

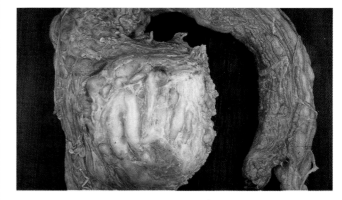

Fig.11.28 Plexiform neurofibroma. This is a major pelvic nerve trunk from a patient with neurofibromatosis and shows gross thickening and expansion by a diffuse tumour. Neurofibromas are benign tumours of nerve sheath origin. They are often seen in von Recklinghausen's neurofibromatosis, an inherited condition which is characterised by café au lait spots, multiple peripheral nerve tumours and is associated with CNS tumours, phaeochromocytoma and an increased risk of developing neurofibrosarcoma.

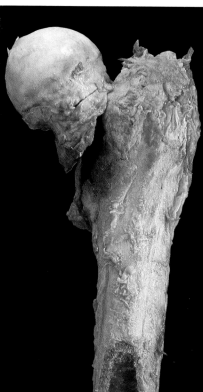

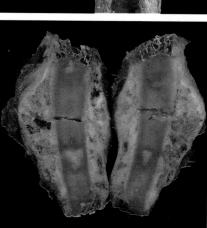

Fig.12.1 Bone fracture. Above, the proximal femur shows an obvious recent subcapital fracture. Part of a rib (below), adjacent to the costochondral junction, shows a transverse fracture, on either side of which is exuberant callus formation. Simple fractures heal by the production of periosteal and then medullary callus, which is followed by new cartilage and bone formation with subsequent re-modelling. The majority of fractures are traumatic in origin but a minority occur through a pre-existent pathological lesion (e.g. a metastasis). Complications include deep venous thrombosis, fat embolism and damage to adjacent tissues (e.g. muscle, tendon, vessels), the latter sometimes leading to Volkmann's contracture.

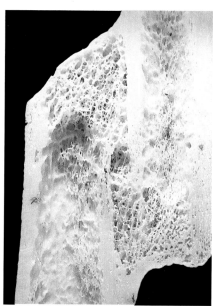

Fig.12.2 Malunion. This macerated segment of a long bone shows clear evidence of a previous fracture but malunion has occurred with deformity resulting from overlap of the bony ends. Malunion follows failure to reduce a displaced fracture. This appearance may also be seen, in a less extreme form, after fracture through an epiphyseal plate (prior to completion of ossification) which results in an abnormal growth pattern.

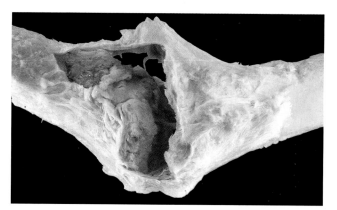

Fig.12.3 Non-union with false joint. Following a fracture of this humerus the bony ends have not been apposed. This has resulted in fibrous union, succeeded by cartilaginous metaplasia and the formation of a pseudarthrosis. Causes of non-union include delayed union (most often due to ischaemia, excessive mobility, local infection or malnutrition), the presence of extraneous tissue between the bone ends or failed treatment of an extensive or widely displaced fracture.

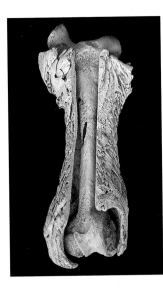

Fig.12.4 Chronic osteomyelitis. The shaft of this macerated femur shows extensive necrosis (the sequestrum) and is surrounded by a dense outer shell of periosteal new bone (the involucrum). Chronic osteomyelitis most often follows an untreated acute episode: this latter is commonest in children and is usually the result of a bacteraemia (often staphylococcal, streptococcal or pneumococcal). *Salmonellae* may be responsible in patients with sickle cell anaemia. Infection commences in the highly vascular metaphysis, most often of a long bone, and is followed by subperiosteal and intramedullary spread.

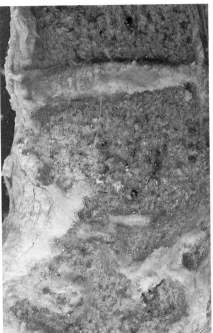

Fig.12.5 Spinal tuberculosis (Pott's disease). This portion of the thoracic spine shows caseous necrosis of two adjacent vertebral bodies with destruction of the intervertebral disc. Tuberculous osteomyelitis, although commonest in long bones, shows a predilection for the spine. It is most often a result of spread from primary pulmonary infection and may be complicated by vertebral collapse, a paravertebral 'cold' abscess or cord compression.

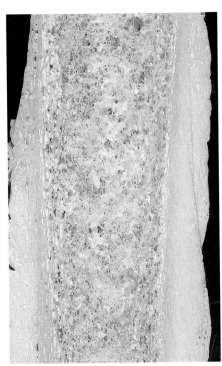

Fig.12.6 Syphilitic periostitis. This is a macerated segment of femur showing a thick layer of subperiosteal new bone. Congenital syphilis classically gives rise to both a florid periostitis (with reactive new bone formation), as in this example, or an osteochondritis (granulomatous inflammation at the ends of long bones). Similar appearances may be seen in tertiary acquired syphilis, in which coexistent gummata may also be present.

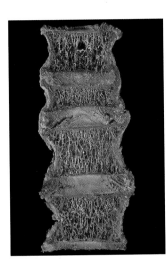

Fig.12.7 Osteoporosis. This macerated section of the lower thoracic and lumbar vertebrae shows a very marked reduction in the amount of cancellous bone associated with a crush fracture. Osteoporosis, defined simply as a decrease in volume of otherwise normal bone, is predominantly a disease of the elderly (particularly females). Causes, other than ageing or the menopause, include prolonged immobility, disuse, Cushing's disease or thyrotoxicosis, but most cases remain idiopathic. The spine and pelvis are most often affected and the principal complication is a fracture.

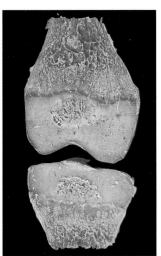

Fig.12.8 Rickets. This section through the lower femur and upper tibia of a child shows marked thickening of the growth plates and a significant failure of endochondral calcification. Rickets and osteomalacia are both characterised by failure of bone mineralisation; the former is a disease of children (prior to completion of growth), while the latter is seen in adults. The commonest cause is diminished serum vitamin D which may be due to dietary deficiency, insufficient sun exposure, malabsorption, chronic renal disease or chronic liver disease. Complications include bony deformities and fractures.

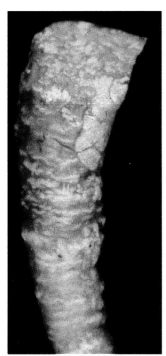

Fig.12.9 Tophaceous gout. This segment of tendon is covered by pale, irregular excrescences (tophi), composed of urate crystals. Gout may be primary, due to an idiopathic disorder of purine metabolism, or secondary, due either to failure of renal urate excretion or excessive turnover of nucleic acids (e.g. in malignant disease or cytotoxic therapy). The consequent hyperuricaemia results in deposition of monosodium urate crystals in joints, periarticular or subcutaneous tissues. Complications include the formation of urate stones in the urinary tract and the deposition of urate crystals in the renal tubules, sometimes leading to renal failure.

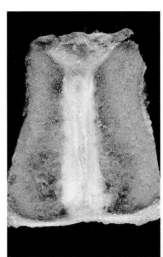

Fig.12.10 Hyperparathyroidism (Osteitis fibrosa cystica). A coronal section through the symphysis pubis shows irregular resorption of the para-articular cortical bone and adjacent hyperaemia. Hyperparathyroidism may be primary, secondary or tertiary (see Chapter 7). Up to 25% of affected patients develop bony changes, characterised by increased bone resorption, medullary fibrosis and the formation of 'brown tumours', which are haemorrhagic foci of fibrosis with cyst formation. In cases secondary to chronic renal failure the features may be modified by coexistent osteomalacia.

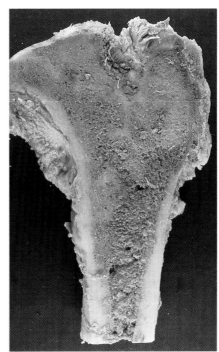

Fig.12.11 Avascular necrosis. This irregular femoral head shows a large, poorly circumscribed area of yellowish necrosis, associated with bony collapse. Avascular necrosis (osseous infarction), which occurs predominantly in the femoral head, most often follows a subcapital fracture. It may also occur in decompression sickness, in patients on steroid therapy, in alcoholics or following renal transplantation. Even though the articular cartilage is spared, microfractures and collapse of the affected bone often lead to arthritis.

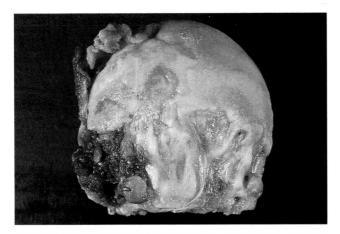

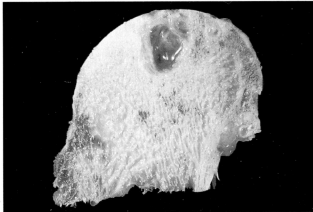

Fig.12.12 Osteoarthrosis. This femoral head (top) is irregular in outline, shows eburnation of its superior aspect and also irregular cystic defects at the sites of cartilaginous loss anteriorly. Below, another example seen in cross-section, shows a multilocular focus of cystic degeneration in the subchondral bone associated with marked osteosclerosis and early osteophyte formation laterally. Osteo-arthrosis is an extremely common, non-inflammatory, 'wear and tear' phenomenon, which affects mainly large weight-bearing joints (usually asymmetrically). Recognised predisposing factors include increasing age, obesity and pre-existent conditions such as congenital hip dislocation, genu varum, Perthes disease or previous fracture. Associated findings in affected patients include cervical spondylosis, hallux rigidus and Heberden's nodes (osteophytes over the terminal interphalangeal joints).

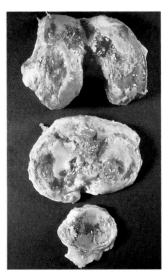

Fig.12.13 Rheumatoid arthritis. The femoral condyles, tibial head and patella show very extensive cartilaginous destruction, particularly at the periphery of the articular surfaces. Osteophytes are absent. Rheumatoid arthritis is a chronic systemic inflammatory disease which is commonest in the 3rd to 5th decades and shows a predilection for females. Small joints are principally affected, usually symmetrically, but progressive involvement of large joints is common. The condition is thought to be autoimmune in nature, is more frequent in patients with HLA-DW4 and is associated with the presence of a serum immunoglobulin known as the rheumatoid factor.

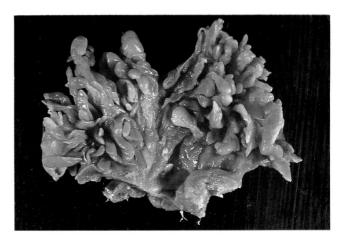

Fig.12.14 Rheumatoid arthritis. This is the synovium from a knee joint, which shows florid synovial villous hyperplasia (pannus formation). Chronic synovial inflammation with hyperplasia are the cardinal features of this disease and precede destruction of the articular cartilage. Systemic features of rheumatoid arthritis may include subcutaneous rheumatoid nodules, splenomegaly, Caplan's syndrome and secondary amyloidosis. Pathologically, the arthritis associated with psoriasis and ulcerative colitis is almost indistinguishable.

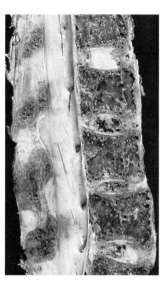

Fig.12.15 Ankylosing spondylitis. A section through these lumbar vertebrae shows widespread osseous fusion through the intervertebral discs, resulting in ankylosis. Ankylosing spondylitis is an idiopathic disorder, which occurs most often in young men and is strongly associated with HLA-B27. The disease is characterised by features similar to those of rheumatoid arthritis, except for the addition of articular ossification. It affects predominantly the axial skeleton. Complications include severe kyphosis, sometimes with respiratory embarrassment.

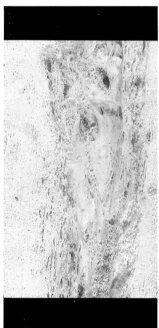

Fig.12.16 Paget's disease (Osteitis deformans). This segment of macerated femur shows marked, irregular thickening of the cortical bone and replacement of cancellous bone by coarse trabeculae. Paget's disease, which is thought to be due to a slow viral infection, affects up to 2% of the population (usually subclinically) and shows a predilection for older adults. It is characterised initially by excessive bone resorption and latterly by a marked increase in irregular new bone formation. The axial skeleton, particularly the spine and skull, is most often affected although the long bones are commonly involved.

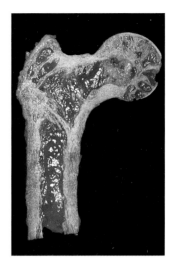

Fig.12.17 Paget's disease. This proximal portion of femur, while showing similar features to Fig. 12.16, also demonstrates residual foci of porotic bone and typical marked hyperaemia. This latter, acting as a multifocal arteriovenous shunt, may give rise to congestive cardiac failure. Other complications of Paget's disease include bony deformity, a predisposition to fractures (the thick but irregular new bone is weaker than normal) and the development of osteosarcoma or chondrosarcoma in 1% of cases.

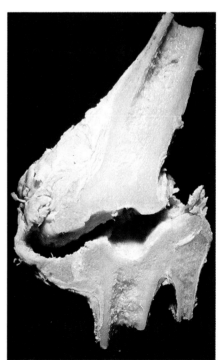

Fig.12.18 Charcot's joint. This coronal section through a knee joint demonstrates gross distortion by subluxation and destruction of the articular cartilage. These features have developed as a complication of neurological disease associated with loss of pain sensation or proprioception. Classical causes include tabes dorsalis, peripheral neuropathy (often diabetic) and syringomyelia.

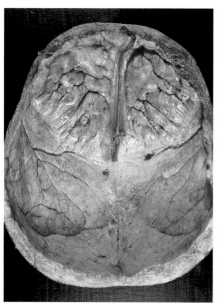

Fig.12.19 Hyperostosis frontalis interna. Projecting from the inner surface of the frontal bones is a well circumscribed mass of extensively ridged, rather greyish bone. Hyperostosis frontalis interna is a not uncommon idiopathic lesion, which is usually seen in late adulthood and is rather more common in women. It is rarely of any clinical significance. Localised reactive hyperostosis of the skull may also sometimes be seen overlying a meningioma.

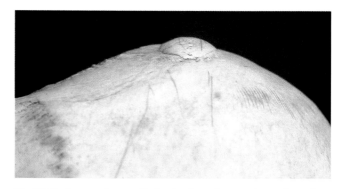

Fig.12.21 Ivory osteoma. Projecting from the superior surface of this skull is a smooth, rounded nodule. Ivory osteomas are benign tumours, composed of densely sclerotic mature bone, which usually arise only from the skull or facial bones. They may present at any age, show a slight predilection for males and never undergo malignant change. They are sometimes a feature of Gardner's syndrome (familial polyposis coli with epidermoid cysts, fibromatoses and bone tumours).

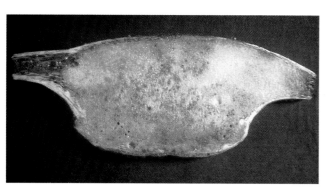

Fig.12.20 Fibrous dysplasia. This segment of rib is markedly expanded by a well circumscribed, pale mass. Fibrous dysplasia is regarded as a hamartomatous lesion, composed of fibrous tissue and woven bone, and may take three forms: (1) the monostotic variant (commonest), which is seen at any age and usually affects long bones or the ribs; (2) the polyostotic variant, which typically presents in childhood, is often unilateral and may also affect the skull; and (3) the polyostotic variant associated with café-au-lait spots and endocrine abnormalities (Albright's syndrome). Sarcomatous change occurs in about 1% of cases.

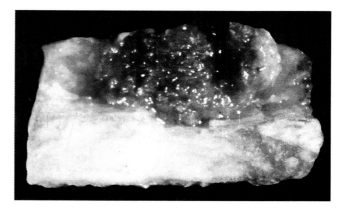

Fig.12.22 Osteoid osteoma. Arising from the cortex of this segment of bone is a well circumscribed, vascular nodule. There is adjacent bony sclerosis. Osteoid osteomas are benign tumours which present most often in childhood or adolescence, are commoner in males and are typically very painful (especially at night). They arise predominantly in the shaft of long bones, particularly the leg, and classically the associated pain is relieved by aspirin. They do not undergo malignant change.

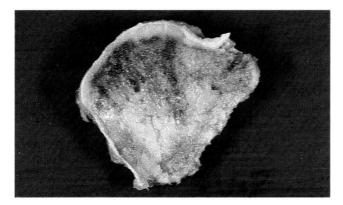

Fig.12.23 Cartilage-capped exostosis. This lesion, which projected from the surface of a femur, shows a pale outer rim of cartilage overlying a nodule of cortical bone. These exostoses (also known as osteochondromas or ecchondromas) are thought to be developmental lesions, derived from laterally aberrant epiphyseal cartilage, which then undergoes endochondral ossification. They present most often in the lower femur or upper tibia of children or young adults. Rarely, they may be multiple (an inherited condition known as diaphyseal aclasis), in which circumstance there is about a 20% risk of developing chondrosarcoma.

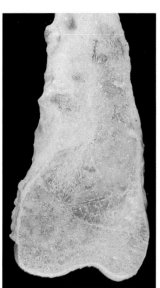

Fig.12.24 Enchondromatosis. This coronal section through the lower end of the femur shows multiple blue-grey nodules of cartilage in the epiphysis, meta-physis and diaphysis. Enchon-dromas are benign tumours, which may be solitary (typically arising in the long bones of young adults) or multiple. The presence of multiple lesions (known as Ollier's disease) is not thought to be hereditary and may be associated with soft tissue haemangiomas (Maffuci's syndrome). Any patient with multiple lesions has a significant risk of developing chondro-sarcoma.

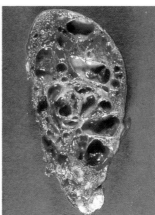

Fig.12.25 Aneurysmal bone cyst. This lesion, removed from the femur, is composed of a well circumscribed haemorrhagic mass within which are numerous vascular spaces. Aneurysmal bone cysts are benign tumours, probably of vascular origin, which typically arise in the long bones or the spine of adolescents and young adults. They are often painful and tend to local recurrence if in-adequately excised. Their occasional coexistence with other adjacent benign tumours of bone further confuses their uncertain histogenesis.

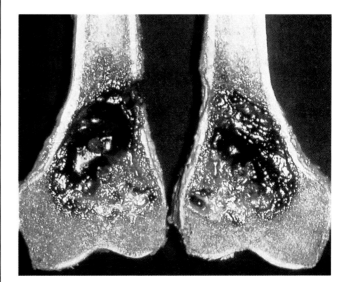

Fig.12.26 Osteoclastoma (giant cell tumour of bone). Arising in the epiphysis of this femur and extending into the metaphysis is a reasonably circumscribed, haemorrhagic mass. Giant cell tumours of bone are uncommon lesions which typically present in young adults and tend to arise in the epiphysis of long bones (particularly in the leg). Their histogenesis is uncertain and they must be dis-tinguished from other giant cell lesions such as chondroblastoma, chondromyxoid fibroma or hyperparathyroidism. Up to 25% behave in a malignant fashion.

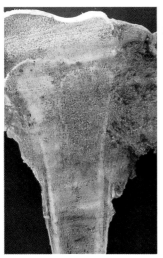

Fig.12.27 Osteosarcoma.
Arising in the metaphysis of this femur is an ill-defined, pale and focally haemorrhagic tumour which has elevated the periosteum and eroded into adjacent soft tissue. Osteosarcoma, in the majority of cases, presents in the first two decades, shows a predilection for males and classically arises in the metaphysis of a long bone (particularly the femur or tibia). A small proportion of cases are seen in the elderly, secondary to Paget's disease (see Figs. 12.16 and 12.17). They tend to extensive local invasion and early haematogenous spread, the overall 5-year-survival being about 20%.

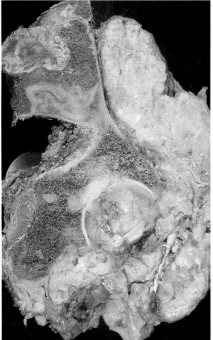

Fig.12.28 Chondrosarcoma.
Arising from the pelvis, adjacent to the acetabulum, is a widely invasive tumour, largely composed of irregularly lobulated, blue-grey cartilaginous tissue. In contrast to osteosarcoma, chondrosarcoma typically presents in the 6th and 7th decades and arises most often in the pelvis (although proximal long bone involvement is not uncommon). It tends to be slow-growing, often attaining a considerable size, and 5-year-survival is about 75%.

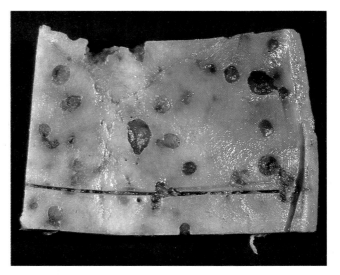

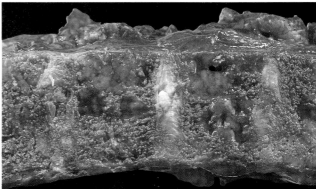

Fig.12.29 Multiple myeloma. This portion of skull (top) shows multiple punched-out lesions containing haemorrhagic tumour. Below, a segment of the spine demonstrates ill demarcated, haemorrhagic, osteolytic lesions in the lower cervical vertebral bodies. Multiple myeloma typically presents in late adulthood and is characterised by a neoplastic proliferation of plasma cells, which classically gives rise to osteolytic lesions in the marrow of the axial skeleton. Excessive immunoglobulin production by the tumour cells allows detection of the light chain Bence-Jones protein in the urine, a useful diagnostic aid. Complications include a predisposition to infection, renal damage and amyloidosis. The prognosis is very variable.

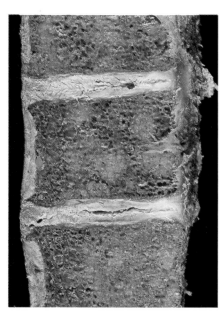

Fig.12.30 Meta-static breast carcinoma. Within the vertebral bodies are scattered, pale, soft necrotic nodules of metastatic tumour. Metastases are the commonest tumour to be found in bone and are most often osteolytic in character. While any disseminated malignancy may involve bone, the commonest primary sources responsible are carcinoma of the breast, lung, prostate, kidney and thyroid.

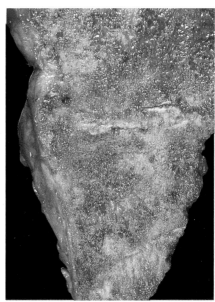

Fig.12.31 Meta-static prostatic carcinoma. The vertebral bodies at the base of this spine are largely replaced by whitish, firm, ill-defined metastatic tumour. Secondary prostatic carcinoma in bone classically stimulates local new bone formation thus giving rise to an osteosclerotic appearance. Breast carcinoma may sometimes have a similar effect.

Index